Joseph M. Strayhorn, Jr. • Kay Yu Yuan Chai
Yanli Zhang-James

The Promise of Psychoeducation in Relieving the Societal Burden of Psychopathology

Springer

Joseph M. Strayhorn, Jr.
Upstate Medical University
Syracuse, NY, USA

Kay Yu Yuan Chai
Upstate Medical University
Syracuse, NY, USA

Yanli Zhang-James
Upstate Medical University
Syracuse, NY, USA

ISSN 3004-9709 ISSN 3004-9717 (electronic)
SpringerBriefs in Modern Perspectives on Disability Research
ISBN 978-981-92-0921-7 ISBN 978-981-92-0922-4 (eBook)
https://doi.org/10.1007/978-981-92-0922-4

This Springer imprint is published by the registered company Springer Nature Singapore Pte Ltd.
The registered company address is: 152 Beach Road, #21-01/04 Gateway East, Singapore 189721, Singapore

SpringerBriefs in Modern Perspectives on Disability Research

Series Editors

This book series on disability research is a comprehensive collection of research on disability and related issues. The series is designed to promote interdisciplinary collaboration and exchange, bringing together scholars and practitioners from different fields to share their perspectives and insights. Disability research is an interdisciplinary field that examines the social, cultural, historical, and political dimensions of disability. It encompasses a wide range of topics, including disability rights, accessibility, assistive technologies, healthcare, education, employment, and social welfare. Disability research scholars employ a range of theoretical and methodological approaches to understand the experiences of people with disabilities, as well as the ways in which disability intersects with other social identities such as race, gender, sexuality, and class.

The series seeks to advance knowledge and understanding of disability by publishing rigorous, innovative, and relevant research. It aims to promote disability rights and social justice by highlighting the ways in which people with disabilities are marginalized and discriminated against in society, and advocating for greater social inclusion and accessibility. The series also seeks to inform policy and practice by disseminating research findings that can help to shape policy decisions and contribute to positive social change.

Human history becomes more and more a race between education and catastrophe.
—H.G. Wells, An Outline of History, 1920

The first step to take is to become aware that love is an art, just as living is an art; if we want to learn how to love we must proceed in the same way we have to proceed if we want to learn any other art, say music, painting, carpentry, or the art of medicine or engineering.
—Erich Fromm, The Art of Loving, 1956

Competing Interests The authors declare the following as potential competing interests: Dr. Strayhorn is director of the Organization for Psychoeducational Tutoring, a nonprofit organization providing psychoeducation. He is the author of several psychoeducational manuals.

Contents

About the Authors

Joseph M. Strayhorn, Jr., M.D. Dr. Strayhorn is Clinical Assistant Professor on the voluntary faculty in the Department of Psychiatry, SUNY Upstate Medical University, Syracuse, New York, and is director of the Organization for Psychoeducational Tutoring (OPT). He appreciates gifts to OPT from Douglas Neff and from the Riley Education Foundation.

Kay Yu Yuan Chai, Ph.D. Dr. Chai is Clinical Assistant Professor, Department of Psychiatry, at SUNY Upstate Medical University, Syracuse, New York.

Yanli Zhang-James, M.D., Ph.D. Dr. Zhang-James is Associate Professor, Department of Psychiatry, at SUNY Upstate Medical University, Syracuse, New York. She has received research support from the National Institute of Mental Health (NIMH), the European Union Horizon 2020 research and innovation program, the American Epilepsy Society, the Carol M. Baldwin Fund of Central New York, SUNY AI funds, and Tris Pharma, Inc.

Chapter 1
Introduction and Definitions

Abstract How can we improve the mental health of the whole population? We define mentally healthy behaviors as those conducive to happiness of both oneself and others; the two goals tend to be positively correlated. We define psychoeducation broadly, as interpersonal influence affecting psychological skills. At present, psychotropic drugs and psychotherapy take center stage regarding methods of improving mental health. This book will argue that straightforward teaching of psychological skills, i.e., psychoeducation (using all the methods that educational science has discovered), has great promise for improving public mental health; it should receive at least as much effort and attention as the other two methods. We will argue that we already have pretty good ideas on which competences constitute mental health, and how to impart them—a major task is scaling what we know. Among the knowledge to be imparted is not only how people can become more mentally healthy themselves, but also how they can create mental-health-friendly environments for others.

Keywords Psychoeducation · Psychological skills · Public mental health · Educational methods · Mental-health-friendly environments · Social determinants

Mental health treatment most often consists of one or both of two major methods: psychopharmacology and psychotherapy. This book promotes a third strategy, psychoeducation, and argues that this could become the most potent instrument in humankind's quest to improve the mental health of the population.

In this book, we're defining "mental health" in a way that is directly tied to the good of society. When we speak of mentally healthy behaviors (including "covert behaviors" of thoughts and emotions), as contrasted with psychopathological ones, we mean those that tend to result in long-term happiness of oneself, and long-term happiness of other people; an important subset is those behaviors that exhibit patience and resilience in coping with the times when happiness eludes us. This definition, unlike some that have been used, does not exclude behaviors that are seemingly rational decisions to be selfish, cruel, or exploitive. Such behaviors have important differences from those that result from psychosis or brain tumors. The

J. M. Strayhorn, Jr. et al., *The Promise of Psychoeducation in Relieving the Societal Burden of Psychopathology*, SpringerBriefs in Modern Perspectives on Disability Research, https://doi.org/10.1007/978-981-92-0922-4_1

person who exploits others and who is dishonest in financial dealings in the course of becoming rich and seemingly enjoying the life of luxury of course has a quite different mental state from the person who is too depressed to get out of bed. But with the definition we are using, neither of these behaviors is mentally healthy. The broad definition of mental health versus psychopathology is meant to subsume the choices which make for a better or worse society. By this broad definition, almost all violent criminal behavior is mentally unhealthy, regardless of whether it qualifies for "not guilty by reason of insanity." The emphasis on behaviors that result in happiness of others as well as of oneself means that the pursuit of mental health and the pursuit of ethical behavior become merged.

Why does the definition of mentally healthy behavior include the effects on happiness of others, as well as the happiness of self? Why merge mental health with ethics? Partly because as a general rule, caring for self and caring for others tend to be positively correlated. Conversely, externalizing problems and internalizing problems are correlated, in the range of $r = 0.3$ to about $r = 0.55$ (Achenbach & Edelbrock, 1984; Krueger, 1999; Caspi et al., 2014; Lahey et al., 2012; Vergunst et al., 2023). Informal observation confirms that at the extremes, criminals tend to be unhappy people, and people who are extremely depressed or anxious on the average tend not to be benefactors of others. The definition of mentally healthy behavior is partly a value judgment, in keeping with centuries-old ethical statements such as the Judeo-Christian "Love thy neighbor as thyself." Similar ideas have been attributed to the Buddha, Hillel, Lao Tzu, Confucius, Immanuel Kant, John Stuart Mill, and various other philosophers.

The above definition applies to behaviors, not to people or their states of being. Any given individual at any time produces behaviors that may differ widely on the scale of mental health. But when referring to a person's state of being, a mentally healthy state denotes both the competences and the circumstances that tend to let the person be happy and help others to be happy, including by using fortitude when necessary. Referring not only to the competences but also circumstances reminds us that mental health strengths or weaknesses do not reside solely within an individual. As an extreme example, if we imagine tremendously psychologically skilled people, and imagine that they are confined and repeatedly tortured, the cruelty toward them surely damages their mental health. Thinking in terms of circumstances as well as competences turns our attention to the necessity for mental-health-friendly environments—a concept we will refer to repeatedly throughout this book. A major goal of psychoeducation, in our broad conception, is teaching people how to create mental-health-friendly environments for others. How to enhance the environments of dyadic relationships, families, friend groups, schools, workplaces, small communities, countries, and even our planet as a whole is included in the bailiwick of psychoeducation.

Psychoeducation is also defined broadly here. We refer to educational methods, for example, instruction, practice, reinforcement, and modeling—any methods meant to enhance learning—which are meant to improve the mental health of the recipients and/or the people they affect. Educational methods of influence also include subtle ones, such as speaking in a way that tends to motivate the person to learn some skill, attributing to the person the ability to learn it, or making the person's surroundings conducive to learning. Psychoeducation can be delivered inadvertently and for the worse, as for example when a parent gives a child what he wants when the child gets angry and aggressive and thus inadvertently teaches aggressive behavior. Psychoeducation for the worse can include the modeling of violence through movies and games meant for entertainment. The term, psychoeducation, has been used more narrowly, to refer to teaching people about a psychiatric disorder they have, and how to cope with it best. Such teaching is a subset of psychoeducation, as we are using the term, but also included are education aimed at primary prevention of disorders that do not exist yet, and education aimed at promoting well-being over and above that subsumed by absence of disorder. The broad definition of psychoeducation subsumes work in what has been called psychological skills training, character education, social and emotional learning, and training in ethics.

Despite our reference to relieving the societal burden of psychopathology in the title of this book, we are sympathetic to the goals of positive psychology. If a person is happy 6 or 7 on a scale of 10, moving to 8 or 9 is a very worthy goal. If people are free of diagnosable disorder, it is a very worthy goal that in addition, they flourish and are benefactors to others. We refer to the burden of psychopathology, though, to emphasize that psychoeducation is not just for the enrichment in the lives of people who are already doing fairly well. We want to remind ourselves that psychoeducation can be aimed with very high priority at prevention or remediation of life-crippling or fatal disorders. What merges goals of positive psychology with those of relief of psychopathology is this: unlike drug treatment, psychoeducation can usually apply the same methods for promoting flourishing as for relieving suffering. For example, becoming competent at social skills including conversation and joint decision-making can not only help relieve social anxiety disorder, depression resulting from loneliness, and the disorders resulting from interpersonal discord, but help elevate the quality of relationships into the supra-normal region. Skills of altering the distribution of self-talk in the direction of more celebration of one's own positive choices and those of others can not only help to relieve depression, but also help continue to make life more pleasant after reaching the non-depressed zone.

How can people be taught, on a large scale, the skills conducive to the happiness of themselves and others, including the skills of creating mental-health-friendly environments? This is not the question primarily dealt with in textbooks of mental health. But, arguably, it is the most important question for society, and has been since antiquity, since society's functioning ultimately is the collective result of decisions by individuals.

This brief book consists of a chain of arguments or claims, the complete documentation of each of which could take up a large book. The short version is this: Advances in psychopharmacology and psychotherapy have not translated into major advances in public mental health. For reasons we will explore, the mental health portfolio and armamentarium need to be enlarged beyond the quest for better medications and more effective psychotherapy. Psychoeducation, because of its greater scalability, holds out potential for greater effects on public mental health. A great deal of accumulated evidence suggests that psychoeducation can be efficacious. However, we are more confident in claiming that psychoeducation *can* produce major positive effects than that it *will* do so.

This book is not "anti" psychopharmacology. It is especially not "anti" psychotherapy, since the psychotherapeutic relationship has been the birthplace of many or most of the effective psychoeducational ideas and methods. We are also not starry-eyed in our predictions of how psychoeducation will change society anytime soon. We will discuss the obstacles to be overcome; we are not holding our breaths waiting for psychoeducation to produce utopia. But we do argue that humanity already has a pretty good idea what competences constitute mental health, and how to teach them; a much wider implementation of such psychoeducation, if skillfully and thoroughly employed, provides hope for society's moving, bit by bit, in a positive direction.

References

Achenbach, T. M., & Edelbrock, C. (1984). Psychopathology of childhood. *Annual Review of Psychology, 35*, 227–256.

Caspi, A., Houts, R. M., Belsky, D. W., Goldman-Mellor, S. J., Harrington, H., Israel, S., Meier, M. H., Ramrakha, S., Shalev, I., Poulton, R., & Moffitt, T. E. (2014). The p factor: One general psychopathology factor in the structure of psychiatric disorders? *Clinical Psychological Science, 2*(2), 119–137.

Krueger, R. F. (1999). The structure of common mental disorders. *Archives of General Psychiatry, 56*(10), 921–926.

Lahey, B. B., Van Hulle, C. A., Singh, A. L., Waldman, I. D., & Rathouz, P. J. (2012). Higher-order genetic and environmental structure of common psychopathology in childhood and adolescence. *Archives of General Psychiatry, 69*(9), 905–915.

Vergunst, F., Tremblay, R. E., Galéra, C., Nagin, D. S., Vitaro, F., & Côté, S. M. (2023). Association of childhood externalizing, internalizing, and comorbid symptoms with long-term outcomes. *JAMA Network Open, 6*(1), e2250920.

Chapter 2
The Societal Burden of Psychopathology: Winning Battles But Losing the War?

Abstract Mental health treatment is more available than it has ever been before. And more is known now, than ever before, about how to conduct such treatment effectively. Research output is prodigious. Yet, by a number of indicators, the mental health of the population has not improved in recent decades, or has even worsened. Indicators include prevalences of disorders and symptoms, suicide and homicide rates, deaths of despair, rates of school shootings and other mass homicides, and fear of one's fellow humans when walking alone. Indicators among young people include surveys of college students, responses to psychological tests, teachers' descriptions of students' behaviors, and rates of psychiatric hospitalizations. The insufficient public health effect of improved clinical methods motivates a quest for methods that can effectively help a much larger segment of the population than clinical mental health services can reach.

Keywords Public mental health · Indicators · Deaths of despair · Depression rates · Suicide rates · Prevalence

Scientific output in the mental health field, over the last century, has been truly prodigious. The American Psychological Association's journal database, PsychInfo (APA, 2026), as of this writing comprises about 2400 journals and about 6 million articles. Research activity in mental health has borne enormous fruit. The understanding of brain functioning has grown by leaps and bounds. The science of psychotropic drug development has moved from accidental discoveries to those based on understanding of brain mechanisms. The US Food and Drug Administration issued 118 approvals of drugs for psychiatric disorders in the 15 years between 2008 and 2023 alone (IsHak et al., 2024). (This is not the number of distinct molecules; we estimate that about 70 distinct psychotropic drugs have been approved to date.) The drugs in current use are more efficacious, less dangerous in overdose, and less addictive than those resorted to in the past.

The field of psychotherapy, like that of psychopharmacology, has been transformed with enormous benefit by the refinement of outcome research. Psychotherapy

J. M. Strayhorn, Jr. et al., *The Promise of Psychoeducation in Relieving the Societal Burden of Psychopathology*, SpringerBriefs in Modern Perspectives on Disability Research, https://doi.org/10.1007/978-981-92-0922-4_1

has moved from an enterprise where one method fits all, to one where specific techniques are tailored for aggression, obsessive compulsive disorder, depression, phobias, panic disorder, insomnia, and others. Psychotherapy has moved, perhaps not completely, from a question of what method has the most charismatic guru advocating it, to the question of what method produces replicable positive outcomes for a specific type of problem.

And, as treatment for mental health conditions has become more evidence-based, it has become more widely employed. In the USA, "Prevalence of 12-month treatment for emotional problems was 12.2% in 1990–2 and 20.1% in 2001–3" (Kessler et al., 2005). And since the turn of the millennium, mental health treatment in the USA has continued to increase steadily (Substance Abuse and Mental Health Services Administration, 2003, 2025).

Mental health treatment has become increasingly destigmatized. As one indicator and perhaps a contributor to this trend, more celebrities have been unafraid to speak publicly about mental health efforts (Galdo, 2025).

Thus, mental health treatments are getting better, and, at least in the USA, where statistics are more readily available to us, more people are partaking of them. It would seem, given these two facts alone, that the mental health of US society should be steadily improving. But is it? Or is it even declining? What is happening regarding the societal burden of psychopathology?

There are a number of possible indicators of the mental health of groups of people. The US National Comorbidity Survey (Kessler et al., 2005), after interviews of over 9000 people about psychiatric symptoms, and application of DSM-IV criteria, reported a lifetime prevalence of any disorder as about 46% (Kessler et al., 2005). Thus, diagnosable disorders were not at all rare. But the finding most relevant to the current discussion is that disorders seemed to be getting more prevalent over time, not less. These authors reported: "Lifetime prevalence estimates are higher in recent cohorts than in earlier cohorts and have fairly stable intercohort differences across the life course…The observed cohort effect is at least partly due to substantive rather than methodological factors."

Since the time of the National Comorbidity Survey, has mental health gotten better or worse? One indicator of mental health of groups is their suicide rate. Since the turn of the millennium, the yearly suicide rates in the USA have formed an almost monotonically increasing function, beginning at 10.4 per 100,000 in 2000 and reaching 14.1 per 100,000 in 2023 (Centers for Disease Control, 2025).

Liu et al. (2020) reported data from the Global Burden of Disease Study that the global incidence of depression increased by about 50% during the time between 1990 and 2017.

"Deaths of despair" have been defined as the sum of deaths due to suicide, drugs, and alcohol. According to reports by the US Congress Joint Economic Committee (2019), such deaths have increased, as scientific progress has attempted to combat them. Rates per 100,000 increased from a little over 15 in the 1950s, to about 23 in 2000, to about 45 in 2017.

Rates of incarceration are a function of several factors, including swings of political sentiment, and are not a great index for the prosocial versus antisocial behaviors in the society as a whole. Nonetheless, it's worth noting that as of year-end 2020, about 1 in 47 US adults was under some form of correctional supervision—incarceration, parole, probation (Kluckow & Zeng, 2022)—and as of spring 2024, about 1.8 million were incarcerated (Vera Institute of Justice, 2024).

The Gallup polling organization in the USA has for several decades tracked answers to the following question: "Is there any area near where you live—that is, within a mile—where you would be afraid to walk alone at night?" In 2023, 40% of respondents answered "yes"; this was the highest rate in 30 years (Saad, 2023).

Deaths by homicide are another indicator of antisocial or externalizing behavior. From the turn of the millennium until recently, the rates of homicide in the USA have remained fairly steady in the range of 5 to 7 deaths per 100,000. Rates increased sharply during the pandemic, but fell afterward to what appears to be about 4.3 per 100,000 in 2025; these rates are about the same as recorded in the mid-1950s, and much lower than the peak in the 1970s, 1980s, and 1990s (Horpedahl, 2026). The rates are affected by demographics, particularly the population fraction of young adult males, the segment most prone to homicide. Among US residents of age 15–34, accidents are the number one cause of death, with suicide and homicide fairly close to one another in second and third place (Centers for Disease Control, 2026). Overall, it's difficult to make inferences about changes in population mental health from this indicator, but we have not arrived at acceptable levels of homicide, if such levels can even be said to exist.

Although homicides are not increasing in recent years, anxiety about school violence has skyrocketed, because of a dramatic increase in school shootings. In the late 1960s, such incidents were 10 or fewer per year; up until 2010 there were usually under 50 incidents per year; from 2016 to 2025, the rates increased to 233 per year, peaking in 2023 at 352 such incidents (Riedman, 2025; Rapa et al., 2024).

Loneliness is gaining widespread attention as a public health problem, conducive to a wide variety of mental health conditions, and has been referred to as an epidemic. Data from 113 countries established that the problem is prevalent, with significant variation between countries (Surkalim et al., 2022). At least in the USA, England, and Mediterranean Europe, loneliness appears to be increasing over time (Infurna et al., 2024).

As the National Comorbidity Study suggested, mental health seems to be getting worse among younger cohorts in the USA. The Healthy Minds Survey samples US college students; the 2024–2025 report (Eisenberg et al., 2025) sampled about 85,000 students from 135 colleges or universities. Thirty-seven percent reported moderate or severe depression; 33% had moderate or severe anxiety. Eleven percent during the previous year had suicidal ideation; 5% made a suicidal plan, and 2% made a suicide attempt. These rates are dramatically higher than those of 2013.

A study by Twenge et al. (2019) reported that the rates of past-year major depressive episodes "increased 52% 2005-2017 (from 8.7% to 13.2%) among adolescents aged 12 to 17 and 63% 2009-2017 (from 8.1% to 13.2%) among young adults 18-25. Serious psychological distress in the last month and suicide-related outcomes (suicidal ideation, plans, attempts, and deaths by suicide) in the last year also increased among young adults 18-25 from 2008-2017 (with a 71% increase in serious psychological distress)."

Twenge et al. (2010) reported on changes in college students' and high school students' MMPI scores over 7 decades: "The current generation of young people scores about a standard deviation higher (average d=1.05) on the clinical scales, including Pd (Psychopathic Deviation), Pa (Paranoia), Ma (Hypomania), and D (Depression). Five times as many now score above common cutoffs for psychopathology..." (p. 145). If the MMPI is a valid indicator of mental health, the mental health of such students appears to have worsened even as more knowledge about mental health has blossomed. Selection factors are possible confounds for these results. The authors believe that cultural shifts best explain the changes.

As an indicator of the mental health of K-12 students, we can examine teachers' reports of their behavior. According to a Pew Foundation Survey of US teachers (Lin et al., 2024):

68% of teachers have experienced verbal abuse from students;
21% say they receive verbal abuse several times/month;
40% have experienced physical violence from students;
58% address students' behavioral issues every day.

Changes in mental health of youth over time are not limited to the USA. In England, rates of admission to hospital wards for mental health concerns and for other reasons have been studied over the time from 2012 to 2022 by Ward et al. (2025). Increases in mental health admissions are significantly larger than those for other reasons. Among children 11–15, the admission rate doubled over that time; for other age groups, the rate increased in the 30–40% range.

To summarize, though mental health clinical treatment has advanced greatly over the last few decades, public mental health itself, by several indicators, seems to have declined over time. Some of the apparent increase in mental health problems may reflect improved detection, clearer diagnostic criteria, and greater public awareness of mental illness; however, these factors alone are unlikely to account fully for the trends described above. What are we to make of this? One explanation is obvious: there are many determinants of mental health that clinicians have no control over. Mental health clinicians can't control electronic media influences, income inequality, availability of jobs, norms regarding drug and alcohol use, the rise or fall of institutions that create social connection, the degree of violence prevailing in neighborhoods, pandemics, decisions about warfare, and other environmental influences that we will explore more later. Less obvious explanations have to do with limitations on how much societal good can be done by drugs and psychotherapy, which we will soon explore in detail. But first we will explore the basic sets of causes of mental health and mental disorder, and relationships between these sets.

References

American Psychological Association. (2026). *PsycInfo*. https://www.apa.org/pubs/databases/psycinfo/

Centers for Disease Control and Prevention. (2025). *Suicide data and statistics*. https://www.cdc.gov/suicide/facts/data.html

Centers for Disease Control and Prevention. (2026). *11 leading causes of death, United States, 2023*. https://wisqars.cdc.gov/lcd

Eisenberg, D., Lipson, S. K., et al. (2025). *The healthy minds study: 2024–2025*. The Healthy Minds Network. https://healthymindsnetwork.org/wp-content/uploads/2025/09/2024-2025_HMS-National-Data-Report_Student.pdf

Galdo, J. (2025). *Celebrities that are speaking out about mental health*. Atlanta Center for Mental Health. https://www.atlmentalhealth.com/post/celebrities-that-are-speaking-out-about-mental-health

Horpedahl, J. (2026). *The US homicide rate in 2025 may have been the lowest ever*. https://economistwritingeveryday.com/2026/01/28/the-us-homicide-rate-in-2025-may-have-been-the-lowest-ever/

Infurna, F. J., Dey, N. E. Y., Gonzalez Avilés, T., Grimm, K. J., Lachman, M. E., & Gerstorf, D. (2024). Loneliness in midlife: Historical increases and elevated levels in the United States compared with Europe. *American Psychologist, 80*(5), 744–756. https://doi.org/10.1037/amp0001322

IsHak, W. W., et al. (2024). *Overview of approved psychiatric medications 2008–2023: A systematic review. World Journal of Advanced Research and Reviews*. https://wjarr.com/sites/default/files/WJARR-2024-0705.pdf

Kessler, R. C., Berglund, P., Demler, O., Jin, R., Merikangas, K. R., & Walters, E. E. (2005). Lifetime prevalence and age-of-onset distributions of DSM-IV disorders in the National Comorbidity Survey Replication. *Archives of General Psychiatry, 62*(6), 593–602.

Kluckow, R., & Zeng, Z. (2022). *Correctional populations in the United States, 2020—Statistical tables*. U.S. Department of Justice, Bureau of Justice Statistics.. https://bjs.ojp.gov/content/pub/pdf/cpus20st.pdf

Lin, L., Parker, K., & Horowitz, J. (2024). *What's it like to be a teacher in America today?* Pew Research Center. https://www.pewresearch.org/social-trends/wp-content/uploads/sites/3/2024/04/ST_24.04.04_teacher-survey_report.pdf

Liu, Q., He, H., Yang, J., Feng, X., Zhao, F., & Lyu, J. (2020). Changes in the global burden of depression from 1990 to 2017: Findings from the Global Burden of Disease Study. *Journal of Psychiatric Research, 126*, 134–140.

Rapa, L. J., Katsiyannis, A., Scott, S. N., et al. (2024). School shootings in the United States: 1997–2022. *Pediatrics, 153*(4), e202306431. https://doi.org/10.1542/peds.2023-06431

Riedman, D. (2025). *K–12 school shooting database*. https://k12ssdb.org/all-shootings

Saad, L. (2023). *Personal safety fears at three-decade high in US*. https://news.gallup.com/poll/544415/personal-safety-fears-three-decade-high.aspx

Substance Abuse and Mental Health Services Administration. (2003). *Results from the 2002 national survey on drug use and health: National findings* (DHHS Publication No. SMA 03–3836). Office of Applied Studies. https://www.ojp.gov/ncjrs/virtual-library/abstracts/results-2002-national-survey-drug-use-and-health-national-findings

Substance Abuse and Mental Health Services Administration. (2025). *Highlights for the 2024 National Survey on Drug Use and Health*. Center for Behavioral Health Statistics and Quality. https://www.samhsa.gov/data/sites/default/files/NSDUH%202024%20Annual%20Release/2024-nsduh-nnr-highlights.pdf

Surkalim, D. L., Luo, M., Eres, R., Gebel, K., van Buskirk, J., Bauman, A., & Ding, D. (2022). The prevalence of loneliness across 113 countries: Systematic review and meta-analysis. *BMJ, 376*, e067068. https://doi.org/10.1136/bmj-2021-067068

Twenge, J. M., Gentile, B., DeWall, C. N., Ma, D., Lacefield, K., & Schurtz, D. R. (2010). Birth cohort increases in psychopathology among young Americans, 1938–2007: A cross-temporal meta-analysis of the MMPI. *Clinical Psychology Review, 30*(2), 145–154. https://doi.org/10.1016/j.cpr.2009.10.005

Twenge, J. M., Cooper, A. B., Joiner, T. E., Duffy, M. E., & Binau, S. G. (2019). Age, period, and cohort trends in mood disorder indicators and suicide-related outcomes in a nationally representative dataset, 2005–2017. *Journal of Abnormal Psychology, 128*(3), 185–199. https://doi.org/10.1037/abn0000410

U.S. Congress Joint Economic Committee. (2019). *Long-term trends in deaths of despair*. https://www.jec.senate.gov/public/index.cfm/republicans/2019/9/long-term-trends-in-deaths-of-despair

Vera Institute of Justice. (2024). *In spring 2024, 1.8 million people were incarcerated in the United States*. https://trends.vera.org

Ward, J. L., Vázquez-Vázquez, A., Phillips, K., Settle, K., Pilvar, H., Cornaglia, F., Gibson, F., Nicholls, D., Roland, D., Mathews, G., Roberts, H., Viner, R. M., & Hudson, L. D. (2025). Admission to acute medical wards for mental health concerns among children and young people in England from 2012 to 2022: A cohort study. *The Lancet Child & Adolescent Health, 9*(2), 112–120. https://doi.org/10.1016/S2352-4642(24)00333-X

Chapter 3
Three Sets of Causes and Remedies for Mental Health and Mental Disorder

Abstract What causes people to behave in a mentally healthy way, or not? We can divide influences into three sets: biology, learning, and situations/environment. For optimum functioning, we need to have a well-functioning nervous system, good habits of responding to situations, and a good environment furnishing us situations to respond to. These sets of influences do not stay separate, but influence one another. Favorable new learning can override some biological dispositions (as for example when people genetically disposed to anxiety learn anti-anxiety techniques); bad learned habits or dangerous environments can result in biological damage to the nervous system (as for example with brain damage from aggressive encounters or drug abuse). Importantly, one person's learned habits become another person's environment. People's habits of criticism, jealousy, verbal or physical abuse, and threatened or actual abandonment, versus kindness, rational joint decision-making, and loyalty, create emotional climates that can be very toxic or very favorable to the mental health of the people they affect. The implication is that widespread learning of psychologically skillful patterns also favorably affects both environmental and biological influences.

Keywords Biological influence · Learning · Environmental factors · Situational factors · Causes of psychopathology · Curative influences · Healing methods

3.1 Biology, Learning, and Situations

What makes people's mental health better, and what makes it worse? We can think of three sets of causes: biological, learning-based, and situational/environmental.

Suppose there is a task that we want a computer to do—analyze data and tell us the result of the analysis, for example. There are three ways that things could go wrong: problems with the hardware, the software, or the input, from the keyboard or elsewhere. Similarly, there are three ways to fix a problem: fix the hardware,

J. M. Strayhorn, Jr. et al., *The Promise of Psychoeducation in Relieving the Societal Burden of Psychopathology*, SpringerBriefs in Modern Perspectives on Disability Research, https://doi.org/10.1007/978-981-92-0922-4_1

revise the software, or improve the input to make it easier for the hardware and software to process successfully.

Here's the analogy to human functioning: there are three ways that people can malfunction behaviorally (including thoughts, emotions, and physiological reactions as types of "behaviors," broadly defined). There can be something wrong with the brain itself. For example, lead toxicity, too much or too little thyroid hormone, injury from brain trauma, autoimmune brain illness, brain tumor, genetically determined brain disorder, drug intoxication or withdrawal state, and infectious illness affecting the brain are a few of the causes of malady that seem to fall under the rubric of biological insults, biomedical causes. When we directly alter the influences upon the brain, by treating an infection, giving a drug thought to change neurotransmission for the better, operating upon a tumor, shutting off the source of a toxic chemical, or altering the level of a hormone for the better, we are making a biological intervention. All these are analogous to hardware issues with the computer.

The second set of causes of people's malfunction is learning-based. For example, a person has learned to use severely critical self-talk, to fear social interaction, to be distrustful and suspicious of other human beings by default, or to expect much of others that they continually disappoint. Or, the person has not learned to modulate the expression of anger, or to delay gratification in the service of goal attainment. These are only a few of many possible examples. And the best remedy for these is more favorable learning: learning to revise maladaptive automatic thoughts and replace them with more adaptive ones; learning new associations between situations and emotions that are preferable to have; learning skills of handling situations well. These are the sorts of learnings that psychotherapy seeks to furnish, and that preventive psychoeducation seeks to furnish to prevent disorders from becoming manifest. Our learnings of how to respond to the inputs from our environments are analogous to computer software.

And just as computers with well-functioning hardware and software aren't capable of delivering good results if the input from the keyboard or other input device is faulty, there are some situations that almost no one can respond to without anguish. There are many other situations that particular people have great difficulty handling. For most human beings, being in deadly combat situations for an extended time, if one survives them, exceeds such capacity. But more common situational influences toward malady include critical, hostile emotional climates, situations where the demands of the situation significantly exceed the person's skill levels, temptations toward pleasurable but harmful experiences (such as those of drug use), unemployment, poverty, bullying, coercion versus freedom, and others. And situational remedies, when they can be employed, include interventions such as removing a child from an abusive environment, shifting a student to a classroom where the demands are more in keeping with abilities, escaping from an environment that values antisocial behavior over productivity, finding a peer group with positive values, and others.

Thinking in terms of these sets of causes is not new. One of us wrote of these sets of causes in a textbook of general psychiatry published several decades ago (Strayhorn, 1981). These sets of causes correspond fairly closely to the "biopsychosocial" model written about by Engel in 1977 and 1980 (and written about by Wade and Halligan as a "model whose time has come" in 2017).

3.2 The Sets of Causal Factors Influence One Another

Life is not so simple that these three sets of causes stay separate from one another. Causal factors from one group very frequently cascade into causes from another group. For example, the environmental circumstance of poverty results in housing with chipping lead paint, which results in the biological problem of lead toxicity. A learned pattern of impulsivity and risk-taking leads to reckless driving, which results in the biological factor of head trauma. Lack of learning of school subjects leads to reduced opportunities for employment in the environment, which in turn leads to gang membership. A learned fear of being overweight leads to the self-starvation of anorexia nervosa, which in turn exerts major biological effects on brain function. A home environment with lots of noisy distractions and constant availability of video games negatively affects social learning and academic learning.

All learning is a biological phenomenon, with the changes learning induces registered somewhere in neurons. It has been exciting when the biological changes induced by learning are visible with current technology. For example, Schwartz et al. (1992) and Baxter et al. (1992) reported finding hyperactivity in the caudate nuclei of patients with obsessive-compulsive disorder, which was normalized by behavioral, nonpharmacological treatment (as well as by pharmacological treatment, as in the second study). Autism is clearly caused by biological factors; one does not learn to be autistic because of family dynamics. But the most effective treatments for autism are learning-based, as exemplified by the classic research of Lovaas (1987) and McEachin et al. (1993). Schizophrenia and bipolar disorder have strong biological contributions from genetics, but a family environment with lots of hostile criticism worsens prognoses for these disorders (Brown et al., 1972; Vaughn & Leff, 1976).

3.3 One Person's Learning Becomes Another's Environment

Some of the environmental events and conditions that negatively impact mental health are acts of nature: hurricanes, earthquakes, lightning bolts, wildfires, droughts, floods. Even with these, people's learned methods of preparedness and their learned decision-making skills may play a big role. But a vast fraction of the environmental conditions that affect our mental health are delivered by other people, and the psychological skills that they have learned or not learned play a huge role in determining our mental health. The upshot of this line of reasoning is that even if we are interested primarily in the strategy of improving mental health by improving the environment, we must wind up using learning-based methods to help people improve the interpersonal environments they present to others.

A major lode of research on the influence of the environment has studied Adverse Childhood Experiences (ACEs). The family environments children are exposed to have been found to exert major effects on mental health variables. To quote Gilgoff et al. (2020):

> At the population level, the Behavioral Risk Factor Surveillance System (BRFSS), which has been collecting abuse and household dysfunction data in up to 42 states and District of Columbia, found that about two-thirds of the US population have been exposed to 1 or more ACEs. The data found ACEs to be associated with the following negative outcomes: traumatic injuries, depression, anxiety, suicide, PTSD, unintended pregnancy, pregnancy complications, fetal death, HIV, sexually transmitted diseases, cancer, diabetes, alcohol and drug abuse, unsafe sex, low educational level (noncompletion of high school), unemployment, and household poverty. Like the ACE Study findings, the BRFSS data showed a graded dose response relationship.

What are ACEs? In the original questionnaire, there were 10: (1) having no one to protect you, (2) loss of a parent, (3) having a mentally ill or suicidal family member, (4) having a family member with a drug problem, (5) violence among adults in the family, (6) a jail or prison term by a family member, (7) verbal abuse toward you, (8) being physically hurt by an adult, (9) feeling unloved, and (10) unwanted sexual contact.

How can we ever reduce or eliminate ACEs? With the exception of loss of a parent through unavoidable illness or injury, all of the ACEs could be reduced if we could somehow increase the psychological skills of the people who interact with children, particularly the skills of kindness, nonviolence, respectful talk, self-care and carefulness, and good decision-making. In other words, a great way to improve the mental health of each generation is to have already improved the mental health of the previous generation. To the extent that the skills of creating a positive emotional climate for children to grow up in are learned skills, the learning of parents and others becomes the environment for the child.

In the study of post-traumatic stress disorder (PTSD), we are reminded of the same principle, that one person's psychological skill repertoire affects the other person's environment. Alisic et al. (2014) reported that the PTSD rate in children and adolescents following "interpersonal trauma" was about 2.5 times as great as that following "non-interpersonal trauma"—about 25% compared with about 10%. In other words, we are more harmed when people do bad things to us than when bad luck strikes. This stands to reason, because that which undermines our ability to trust and to have good will toward our fellow human beings strikes at key aspects of our functioning. And the prevalence of interpersonal trauma is high. As one example, Coker et al. (2016) reported that about a quarter of young adult women had experienced physical violence from a partner, and a similar fraction reported sexual violence from a partner.

Later in this book, we will consider in more detail which learnable skills constitute mental health. We will also tackle more thoroughly the question of what factors constitute a mental-health-friendly environment. For now, we can simplify by realizing that a large fraction of learnable psychological skills are those that result in our being able to get along with others with kindness and good will, and without cruelty and violence; and a large fraction of what constitutes a mental-health-friendly environment is being around people with those same skills.

References

Alisic, E., Zalta, A. K., van Wesel, F., Larsen, S. E., Hafstad, G. S., Hassanpour, K., & Smid, G. E. (2014). Rates of post-traumatic stress disorder in trauma-exposed children and adolescents: Meta-analysis. *The British Journal of Psychiatry, 204*, 335–340. https://doi.org/10.1192/bjp.bp.113.131227

Baxter, L. R., Schwartz, J. M., Bergman, K. S., Szuba, M. P., Guze, B. H., Mazziotta, J. C., Alazraki, A., Selin, C. E., Ferng, H. K., & Phelps, M. E. (1992). Caudate glucose metabolic rate changes with both drug and behavior therapy for obsessive–compulsive disorder. *Archives of General Psychiatry, 49*(9), 681–689.

Brown, G. W., Birley, J. L., & Wing, J. K. (1972). Influence of family life on the course of schizophrenic disorders: A replication. *The British Journal of Psychiatry, 121*, 241–258.

Coker, A. L., Follingstad, D. R., Bush, H. M., & Fisher, B. S. (2016). Are interpersonal violence rates higher among young women in college compared with those never attending college? *Journal of Interpersonal Violence, 31*(8), 1413–1429. https://doi.org/10.1177/0886260514567958

Engel, G. L. (1977). The need for a new medical model: A challenge for biomedicine. *Science, 196*(4286), 129–136.

Engel, G. L. (1980). The clinical application of the biopsychosocial model. *The American Journal of Psychiatry, 137*(5), 535–544.

Gilgoff, R., Singh, L., Koita, K., Gentile, B., & Marques, S. S. (2020). Adverse childhood experiences, outcomes, and interventions. *Pediatric Clinics of North America, 67*(2), 259–273. https://doi.org/10.1016/j.pcl.2019.12.0017

Lovaas, O. I. (1987). Behavioral treatment and normal educational and intellectual functioning in young autistic children. *Journal of Consulting and Clinical Psychology, 55*(1), 3–9.

McEachin, J. J., Smith, T., & Lovaas, O. I. (1993). Long-term outcome for children with autism who received early intensive behavioral treatment. *American Journal on Mental Retardation, 97*(4), 359–372.

Schwartz, J. M., Stoessel, P. W., Baxter, L. R., Martin, K. M., & Phelps, M. E. (1992). Systematic changes in cerebral glucose metabolic rate after successful behavior modification treatment of obsessive–compulsive disorder. *Archives of General Psychiatry, 49*(9), 681–689.

Strayhorn, J. M. (1981). *Foundations of clinical psychiatry*. Year Book Medical Publishers.

Vaughn, C., & Leff, J. (1976). The measurement of expressed emotion in the families of psychiatric patients. *The British Journal of Social and Clinical Psychology, 15*(2), 157–165. https://doi.org/10.1111/j.2044-8260.1976.tb00021.x

Wade, D. T., & Halligan, P. W. (2017). The biopsychosocial model of illness: A model whose time has come. *Clinical Rehabilitation, 31*(8), 995–1004.

Chapter 4
Can Drugs Relieve the Societal Burden of Psychopathology?

Abstract There has been much progress in psychopharmacology in recent decades. But there are some reasons to believe that medications are limited in their abilities to make society mentally healthier. One problem has to do with efficacy. Several meta-analyses have concluded that the advantage over placebo conferred by antidepressants in the treatment of depression, although statistically significant with sizeable samples, is only about 2 points on a 50-point scale. Given the dependence upon randomized controlled trials, much of what we know about efficacy of psychotropic medications is information about what happens in about 12 weeks, but psychiatric conditions tend to be chronic, and medications often need to be maintained for years to treat them; we know little about the long-term effects. However, we do know enough to recognize a problem over and above efficacy: oppositional tolerance. This refers to the tendency of biological systems to oppose the effects of medications, i.e., to downregulate the pathways drugs enhance, and to upregulate the ones they oppose. This can lead to withdrawal effects. Oppositional tolerance, which is a much bigger problem with some drugs than others, can lead to permanent changes, such as those of tardive dyskinesia and supersensitivity psychosis, and it has been hypothesized to worsen the course of psychiatric illness.

Keywords Oppositional tolerance · Efficacy · Antidepressants · Antipsychotics · Benzodiazepines · Withdrawal effects · Long-term effectiveness · Homeostatic changes

There have been many, many studies of the efficacy of psychotropic drugs in the last few decades. We now know vastly more about neurotransmitters, and the effects of increasing or decreasing their action, than we did a few decades ago. There is no doubt that there has been an explosion of knowledge about psychopharmacology since the mid-twentieth century. The professions of psychiatry, and of nurse practitioners in psychiatry, have gradually moved more and more to be professions of "prescribers," with society delegating to psychologists, social workers, and counselors the learning-based psychotherapeutic interventions, and delegating to no

J. M. Strayhorn, Jr. et al., *The Promise of Psychoeducation in Relieving the Societal Burden of Psychopathology*, SpringerBriefs in Modern Perspectives on Disability Research, https://doi.org/10.1007/978-981-92-0922-4_1

particular profession the task of promoting mental-health-friendly environments. There are some who feel that the biological contributions to mental disorders dominate the other causes; these are optimistic that neuroscience and psychopharmacology will provide the ultimate mental health triumphs. Although the future always brings surprises, we predict that psychopharmacology will never, by itself, have the impact on mental health that society needs. We will not be arguing that psychotropic drugs are uniformly harmful, or that they should not be used. Indeed, sometimes they can be life-saving or life-changing for the better.

4.1 What Are Psychotropic Drugs Used For?

If a drug company executive, who is interested only in profit for the company, were offered by a magic genie the knowledge of a chemical that was a miracle cure for any two psychiatric conditions that were picked, what conditions should those be? Surely the answer would be anxiety and depression. In prevalence rates, these two sets of disorders routinely top the list. (They are sometimes rivaled by substance abuse disorders, a large fraction of which are arguably secondary to anxiety and/or depression.) The benzodiazepines climbed to the top of the list of most frequently prescribed drugs in the second half of the twentieth century, because anxious people found that they quickly lowered anxiety. The selective serotonin reuptake inhibitors and the serotonin and norepinephrine reuptake inhibitors have brought in billions of dollars of revenue for drug companies, because they occupy the enviable position of being first-line drug treatments for both depressive and anxiety disorders.

Because they are recommended for anxiety and depression, a significant fraction of the US citizenry takes antidepressant medication. According to the National Health and Nutrition Examination Survey (Brody & Gu, 2020), during 2015–2018, 13.2% of US adults aged 18 and over used antidepressant medications in the past 30 days. Use was higher among women (17.7%) than among men (8.4%). Antidepressant use increased with age—24.3% of women aged 60 and over took antidepressants. From an earlier iteration of the same survey, Pratt et al. (2017) reported the prevalence of long-term use of antidepressants. During 2011–2014, 68.0% of persons aged 12 and over who took antidepressant medication had been taking them for 2 years or more; 21.4% of males and 27.2% of females who took antidepressants had been taking them for 10 years or longer.

Another major candidate for the drug company wish list would be a completely safe and effective sleeping pill. The prevalence of complaints of trouble sleeping is high, and the market for sleeping pills also runs in the billions of dollars (Reports and Data, 2025). A 2023 survey commissioned by the American Academy of Sleep Medicine (2023) reported that 75% of respondents reported at least occasionally ingesting (or inhaling) something—pills (prescription, over the counter, melatonin), alcohol, marijuana—to help them get to sleep.

And a fourth candidate would be a drug for misbehavior—for aggressive, uncooperative, selfish, disruptive, impulsive, undisciplined behavior, in children and adults. The medicines for ADHD, which address a portion of these problems, are among the most efficacious psychotropic drugs known. But treatment of ADHD can alleviate only a very small fraction of human bullying, cruelty, verbal abuse, sexual abuse, exploitation, chronic anger, and hostile interpersonal environments. Such psychopathology has no single diagnosis: one of us catalogued the DSM diagnoses that mentioned anger, hostility, irritability, etc. as possible features; the total came to 52 diagnoses (Strayhorn, 2026). But psychopathology in this realm is especially important, since it tends to create more psychopathology in those who are victims of cruel or hostile behavior.

Interestingly, our imagined profit-seeking drug executive should probably not pick a drug for psychosis, simply because the prevalence rates for psychotic disorders are not as high as the other conditions mentioned. Antipsychotics are given more often for non-psychotic conditions than they are for psychosis. A study of US adults given antipsychotics (Dennis et al., 2020) reported that the number one indication was major depression, with about a third of prescriptions given for that reason. About 16% of antipsychotic prescriptions were for insomnia. In children, the antipsychotics are even more predominantly used for non-psychotic conditions, especially disruptive behavior; only 3–4% of antipsychotic use in children was for schizophrenia or psychosis (Coleman, 2013).

Of interest to our premise about the promise of learning-based intervention, most of the disorders that are "cash cows" for psychopharmacology can also be treated by well-studied learning-based interventions, of demonstrated efficacy. We will more thoroughly discuss later that cognitive behavior therapy for depression has been shown to have a decent effect size in meta-analyses. Desensitization for anxiety has a record of efficacy dating from the mid twentieth century; cognitive behavior therapy for anxiety is effective. For insomnia, rates of improvement for CBT-I, cognitive behavior therapy for insomnia, not only rival but exceed those for sleeping pills. For disruptive behavior, ADHD medications and learning-based interventions have complementary roles, with behavioral intervention, particularly parent training, being efficacious for the portion of misbehavior that is not accounted for by ADHD.

4.2 How Efficacious Is Drug Treatment for Anxiety and Depression?

It is surprising how much the evidence points to the conclusion that the first-line antidepressants, the SSRIs, do not work very well for depression. In a meta-analysis (Jakobsen et al., 2017) which synthesized 131 randomized trials, comprising 27,422 participants:

"SSRIs significantly reduced the Hamilton Depression Rating Scale (HDRS) at end of treatment (mean difference −1.94 HDRS points; 95% CI −2.50 to −1.37; $P<0.00001$; 49 trials.... The effect estimate, however, was below our predefined threshold for clinical significance of 3 HDRS points."

These findings should be unsettling to all who would rely on antidepressants. We have a huge sample size, and 131 different randomized trials. The Hamilton Depression Rating Scale has a range from 0 to 50. An improvement of 2 points on that scale could be accomplished, for example, by a movement in the item on "insight," from denial of depression to acknowledging being depressed and ill, while leaving every other item the same. The "minimal important difference" in the Ham-D is usually felt to be at least 3 points (Hengartner & Plöderl, 2022); this and the use of the HAM-D as the gold standard for depression treatment trials have been debated (Hieronymus et al., 2020). Still, the average improvement of about 2 points is enough to create millions of customers and revenues/expenditures of billions of dollars for drug treatment of depression. In understanding this, it's important to realize that the two-point improvement attributable to medication is over and above that attained with placebo. When taking into account placebo improvement, the improvement the average patient sees is considerably higher.

The Jakobsen et al., 2017 meta-analysis mentioned above also looked at remission rates in studies where the response to SSRIs was dichotomized into remission versus non-remission. This cut down the sample size considerably. For placebo, 510 out of 2003 people remitted, or 25.5%. For SSRI, 781 out of 2211 people remitted, or 35.3%. The difference in remission rates is about 10%, which gives a Number Needed to Treat of 10: that is, you need to treat 10 people, on the average, before there is 1 who responds to the drug but would not have responded to placebo. If we divide 25.5% by 35.3%, we get that about 72% of the people who respond to SSRIs (many of whom will be continued on SSRIs indefinitely) would have remitted on placebo.

How good are the first-line antidepressants in alleviating depression in children and adolescents? A meta-analysis (Cipriani et al., 2016) of SSRIs and SNRIs for 9- to 18-year-olds reported that the 95% confidence interval for the effect size of fluoxetine did not subsume zero, thus meeting criteria for statistical significance. But the lower bound of the confidence interval was an improvement of 0.03 SMD (standardized mean difference) units, for all practical purposes zero. Moreover, the SSRIs with confidence intervals that *did* subsume zero, i.e., with non-significant effect sizes, were all the rest of those studied: duloxetine, venlafaxine, sertraline, citalopram, escitalopram, and paroxetine. Thus, this meta-analysis gives us little confidence that serotonin reuptake inhibition brings relief of depression in 9- to 18-year-olds.

For anxiety, the efficacy story for the SSRIs at first glance appears more favorable. A meta-analysis of SSRI effects on anxiety in adults (Jakubovski et al., 2019) yielded an average standardized mean difference (SMD) effect of 0.60, where 0.5 is taken as a moderate effect size and 0.8 as a large one; the SNRI average effect size was 0.51. But a meta-analysis by Slee et al. (2019) reported effect sizes in terms of number of points improvement on the Hamilton Anxiety Scale (range 0 to 56) that are reminiscent of those for depression: e.g., for some SSRIs, 2.5 points for escitalopram, 2.4 for fluoxetine, 2.9 for sertraline; for some SNRIs, 3.1 for duloxetine, and 2.7 for venlafaxine. For children, according to the Child/Adolescent Anxiety Multimodal Study (CAMS, summarized by Nicotra & Strawn, 2023), the addition of sertraline to cognitive behavior therapy increased the response rate from about 60% to about 81%. Cognitive therapy alone produced a higher rate of response (60%) than sertraline alone (55%), but the difference was not significant. And the response rate for sertraline is that for getting on the drug and continuing it, perhaps indefinitely, whereas the response rate for CBT is for getting the therapy and not continuing it indefinitely. Several patients have remarked that the SSRIs for them were a "Well, whatever" drug—it made it much easier to think, "Well, whatever" in response to situations that would previously have elicited something more like "Oh no, oh no!" And that movement is often helpful when anxiety is subtracting greatly from life's enjoyment.

Unfortunately, there's another caveat accompanying the demonstrated efficacy of the SSRIs upon anxiety and the "Well, whatever" effect. There is evidence that the SSRIs and SNRIs subtract not only from the distressing emotion of fear, but also from the experience of positive emotions, and thereby reduce motivation; this has been called "SSRI-induced indifference" (Sansone & Sansone, 2010). Price et al. (2009), in a qualitative study of this phenomenon, quoted a number of SSRI recipients. Some of them reported feeling detached from both positive and negative emotions, emotionally numb, unable to feel joy, less connected to people, emotionally distant from significant others. Masdrakis et al. (2023) reviewed 50 studies of this phenomenon—antidepressant-induced emotional blunting or apathy. Studies in this review found prevalences of this phenomenon ranging from 5.8 to 50%. A 2023 review by Barbosa Eyler cited agreement among all reports that the phenomenon occurred more frequently with SSRIs than with other classes of antidepressants. McCabe et al. (2010), using fMRI, studied brain responses to pleasurable stimuli (the sight and taste of chocolate) in healthy volunteers given the SSRI citalopram, versus reboxetine (a selective noradrenaline reuptake inhibitor) or placebo. The citalopram group showed less activation in brain regions producing reward (ventral striatum, ventral medial orbitofrontal cortex) than the other two groups. Most studies on this phenomenon report that it is dose related and that it often disappears upon discontinuation of SSRIs, which tends to confirm that this is a drug side effect and not a symptom of underlying disorder. Most studies also point out that a certain fraction of patients, particularly those whose original emotions were overwhelmingly negative, welcome emotional numbing—the positive emotions were not high to begin with.

4.3 A Knowledge Problem in Psychopharmacology: Short-Term Versus Long-Term

The vast fraction of what we know about drug efficacy, and what drug companies use to prove it, comes from randomized controlled trials subsuming a few weeks to a few months. On the other hand, most psychiatric conditions are chronic, and successful treatment with medications usually requires maintenance treatment for efficacy to continue. Most of the medical and psychological establishment is wedded to randomized studies as the only legitimate source of causal inferences. (This belief has been disputed (Strayhorn, 2021; Glasziou et al., 2007; Smith & Pell, 2003.) But randomized trials can only maintain the separation of participants into groups for a limited time. If a treatment proves superior to another in the short term, the ethics of keeping research participants in the inferior treatment group over the long term are questionable, and in any case, research participants simply don't want to abide by the dictates of researchers over a course of years. The upshot is that randomized trials tell us little about the long-term effects of psychotropic drugs, despite the fact that the long-term effects are the most important piece of information for us to know.

4.4 The Problem of Oppositional Tolerance

There are two mechanisms whereby the favorable short-term effects of a drug can create long-term, perhaps long-lasting or permanent, effects. Let's first discuss a mechanism that leads to a "Hooray for the drug" conclusion. This is the "use it and therefore don't lose it" effect. Using a muscle more, and putting more demands upon it, tends to make it bigger and stronger, and conversely, disuse leads to atrophy. The same phenomenon appears to apply to neurons and neuronal pathways. For example, suppose someone with ADHD is helped by medication to make careful decisions, to organize, to plan, to inhibit impulses, to exert cortical control over limbic-originating emotional signals. According to the use it or lose it theory, the neurons involved in these activities are stimulated to thrive. And indeed, there is some evidence for this effect, from examining cortical thicknesses in people with ADHD treated and untreated with stimulants, as well as non-ADHD comparators (Castellanos et al., 2002; Shaw et al., 2009; Walhovd et al., 2020) but also some evidence against long-term effects of medication on cortical thickness (van der Pal et al., 2024).

It is possible that the same phenomenon occurs for the neuronal pathways that underlie the positive effects of other drugs. There is evidence, for example, that psychosis is not good for the brain, and that antipsychotic drug treatment earlier in a psychotic illness is better than that initiated later (Wyatt, 1991; Catalan et al., 2025). The data seem to indicate that practice by the neural pathways involved in psychosis increases the capability of the brain for producing psychosis.

However, there is another phenomenon in operation the longer psychotropic drugs are given. The word *homeostasis* refers to the tendency of a system to oppose deviations from the initial state, through negative feedback loops. The related term, *oppositional tolerance*, refers to neuronal systems adjusting to a drug that produces a certain change, or perturbation, by producing an opposing effect. For example, oppositional tolerance to a drug that blocks dopamine receptors results in increased sensitivity of dopamine receptors. A drug, such as alcohol or a benzodiazepine, that increases GABA (gamma amino butyric acid) transmission, eventually results in lower GABA activity when the drug is withdrawn (Dharavath et al., 2023; Warlick et al., 2020). The results can include great agitation and anxiety. As another example, cocaine produces its euphoric effects by enhancing dopamine transmission; positron emission tomography (PET) scans have demonstrated, in rhesus macaques, downregulation of dopamine receptors persisting for at least a year after withdrawal from cocaine (Nader et al., 2006), in some, but not all of the animals studied. PET scans in humans have also demonstrated, after withdrawal from cocaine, persistence of dopamine downregulation for at least several months (Volkow et al., 1993). As another example, users of opiates in the beginning of their drug use experience very pleasurable strong stimulation of reward centers, mediated by dopamine; over time, downregulation of reward pathways makes experiences such as eating, sexual activity, or socializing less pleasurable (Garland et al., 2013). The word *tolerance* refers to the fact that the longer the drug is given, the more the oppositional actions reduce the initial effects, and it sometimes requires greater and greater doses to produce the initial effects. And the phrase *withdrawal effects*, with the euphemism *discontinuation syndrome* sometimes substituted, refers to what happens when the person is left with the opposing effects when the drug is discontinued. The word *dependency* describes what people do to avoid withdrawal effects: keep on taking the drug. The word *tachyphylaxis* refers to the drug's losing its efficacy over time.

The history of drug therapy includes a repeated story of great enthusiasm about the effects of a drug, followed by the gradual accrual of evidence for troublesome withdrawal effects. Withdrawal effects of alcohol and opiates have been recognized for at least two or three centuries. Experience with these gave reason to hypothesize that withdrawal from a psychotropic drug can produce the opposite of the effects the drug is meant to have. But over and over, the finding of this phenomenon appears to be surprising. Let's review the problem of oppositional tolerance with a few classes of psychotropic medications. Let's begin with the antidepressants, which are cornerstones of psychopharmacology, being first line drugs for anxiety, depression, and obsessive-compulsive disorder.

4.5 Antidepressants

The SSRIs (selective serotonin reuptake inhibitors) took over the antidepressant market beginning with the introduction of fluoxetine in 1987; the SSRIs had the huge advantage over the tricyclic antidepressants of being much safer in overdose. But then the evidence for an SSRI withdrawal syndrome (a.k.a. discontinuation syndrome) began to accumulate (Glenmullen, 2000).

Can the homeostatic changes in response to the antidepressants result, in the long term, in more depression, not less? There is evidence that this is the case. According to Cosci and Fava (2021):

> Behavioral toxicity related to antidepressant drugs may be explained on the basis of the oppositional model of tolerance: continued drug treatment may recruit processes that oppose the initial acute effects of a drug. This may explain loss of treatment efficacy….

> These processes may also propel the illness to a more malignant and treatment-unresponsive course .... Oppositional processes ... may [result] in the appearance of new withdrawal symptoms, rebound symptomatology, persistent postwithdrawal disorders. In the long run, antidepressants may increase chronicity, vulnerability to depressive disorders, and comorbidity. The number of clinical studies supporting the oppositional model of tolerance has progressively increased over the years.

And as Fava (2020) puts it:

> The oppositional model of tolerance may explain loss of treatment efficacy during maintenance treatment... These processes may also direct the illness into a treatment-unresponsive course.... When drug treatment ends, oppositional processes no longer encounter resistance, resulting in potential onset of new withdrawal symptoms, persistent post-withdrawal disorders, ... and resistance to treatment if it is reinstituted. In all these cases, antidepressant medications may constitute a form of iatrogenic comorbidity, which increases chronicity and vulnerability to depressive episodes.

One way of testing the hypothesis that the antidepressants induce oppositional tolerance that can worsen the course of depression was employed by Andrews et al. (2011). These investigators meta-analyzed randomized trials that followed up participants until medication withdrawal. The study compared the rates of relapse of depression when responders to medication were taken off medication, with the rates of relapse when responders to placebo were taken off placebo. The hypothesis: "the buildup of oppositional tolerance during ADM [antidepressant medication] treatment will attempt to bring monoamine levels back to equilibrium, which will cause them to overshoot the equilibrium after ADM treatment is discontinued." The test: "Patients who remit with ADM treatment will have a higher risk of relapse after treatment stops than patients who remit without ADM treatment." The results: Placebo remitters had an average 25% rate of relapse after discontinuation of placebo. SSRI remitters had an average relapse rate of 49%, and SNRI [serotonin and norepinephrine reuptake inhibitors) remitters had an average relapse rate of 42%.

One might criticize this study by arguing, "The drug remitters were the ones who really needed the drug, whereas the placebo remitters were selected for not needing the drug. That's why the drug remitters relapsed more often." But we can recall the meta-analysis referred to earlier, with a conclusion that 72% of the SSRI remitters would have remitted with placebo. The difference in remission rates between drug and placebo in that meta-analysis was only about 10%, whereas the difference in relapse rates upon withdrawal in the Andrews study was 24% for SSRIs.

In addition, Andrews et al. reported the following:

> As discussed above, the lower relapse rate of the PBO group could be due to a selection bias problem.... To formally test this, we included as covariates the minimum number of depressive episodes required for entry into the study, whether treatment resistant patients were targeted, and the dropout rate during the acute treatment phase. None of the sample characteristic variables were significant, while the treatment variable remained significant, β=0.342, SE=0.080, p=0.0001. The inclusion of other covariates also did not influence the significance of this variable.

The uncomfortable idea this study suggests is that the ill effects of coming off SSRIs or SNRIs are greater than the positive effects of going on them in the first place.

The Andrews et al. meta-analysis was based on randomized clinical trials, which have limited time of exposure to SSRIs or SNRIs. How can we study the effects of withdrawal from antidepressants that have been given for years? Cohen et al. (2006) studied the effects of withdrawal of antidepressants from pregnant women. Of those who withdrew from their medications, the rate of relapse into depression was a disturbingly large 68%. Of those who maintained their medication, the rate of relapse was 26%. The difference is 42%, yielding a number needed to treat of 2.4. By contrast, the number needed to treat to obtain remission in the Jakobsen et al. meta-analysis was 10, and the percent difference was 10%. Again, the idea suggested is that coming off antidepressants is much more "effective" at producing relapse than going on them is, in producing remission. This finding would be expected if oppositional tolerance makes the individual more vulnerable to depression when medications are withdrawn.

The notion that quite unpleasant withdrawal symptoms from antidepressants can be protracted or permanent was supported by a study by Hengartner and Plöderl (2022). These researchers obtained data from people who participated in an Internet forum on antidepressants and withdrawal from them. The sample included long-term users: the mean time on antidepressants was 96 months, or 8 years. The top of the range was greater than 20 years. In this sample, the mean duration of withdrawal symptoms was 37 months. Throughout the withdrawal experience, affective symptoms, mostly anxiety, depression, emerging suicidality, and agitation, were reported by 81%. Somatic symptoms, mostly headache, fatigue, dizziness, brain zaps, visual changes, muscle aches, tremor, diarrhea, and nausea, were reported by 75%. Sleep problems (44%) and cognitive impairments (32%) were mentioned less frequently.

Read (2020) gathered data on a convenience sample of long-term users of antidepressants who were trying to discontinue them or had discontinued them. "The majority (59%) had taken antidepressants for more than 3 years. Of those who were still taking them, 29% had been doing so for at least 20 years. Sixty-one percent reported some degree of withdrawal effects, and 44% of these described the effects as 'severe.'" The symptoms included anxiety/panic (66%), irritability (62%), dizziness (44%), brain zaps (43%), nightmares (37%), and nausea (35%). Duration of treatment was related to severity of withdrawal.

By contrast, a study by Henssler et al. (2024) estimated the prevalence of withdrawal effects with antidepressants to be much lower: "Subtracting non-specific effects, we estimate the frequency of antidepressant discontinuation symptoms to be in the range of approximately 15%, thus affecting about one in six to seven patients. Evidence that about one in 35 patients suffers from severe antidepressant discontinuation symptoms must be considered preliminary at present…." But the Henssler et al. study was a meta-analysis from randomized clinical trials. The duration of treatment before withdrawal was reported to range from 1 to 156 weeks—in other words, with a maximum of 3 years. The durations of treatment reported by Hengartner and Read were much longer. Moncrieff et al. (2025) reanalyzed the Henssler et al. data including only studies that specifically asked participants about withdrawal symptoms, and found a higher incidence; these authors also noted the short duration of antidepressant exposure.

The phenomenon of "brain zaps," or sudden sensations as if electricity were going through the head, is a distinctive feature of SSRI and SNRI withdrawal. Papp & Onton (2022) gathered a sample of 2267 people who reported brain zaps as a withdrawal effect of these drugs. Most said that the brain zaps had a negative effect on quality of life. Eight hundred forty-four respondents reported zaps whenever they skipped a dose of medication. The latency of onset was proportional to the half-life of the SSRI. About 2/3 of respondents restarted medications to get rid of zaps, and this helped in 89%. Less than a third told the prescriber about these.

Another persisting side effect after SSRI withdrawal has been called PSSD, post-SSRI sexual dysfunction. According to Peleg et al. (2022):

> PSSD can emerge after brief or long-term exposure to SSRIs and can persist for months, years, or indefinitely. It affects both genders, and currently there is no established treatment. The incidence and prevalence of this condition is not known. Rat studies have demonstrated a permanent reduction in the sensitivity of 5HT1A receptors following the discontinuation of fluoxetine. Moreover, studies of the chronic use of SSRIs in very young rodents resulted in a sustained reduction in sexual behavior in adulthood .....We propose that down-regulation of the pre-synaptic autoreceptors is part of the underlying mechanism of PSSD. (p. 92)

While the mechanism of post-SSRI sexual dysfunction is not fully known, it is plausible that it results from downregulation of serotonin receptors in an example of homeostatic effects. In humans, we might theorize that lasting effects on sexual function could be explained psychologically, by a vicious cycle of self-consciousness induced by acute effects. However, such an explanation is hardly plausible for rats. And the demonstration of *permanent* reduction in 5HT1A receptors must disrupt the belief that untoward side effects of these medications can always be reversed with discontinuation.

If withdrawal from antidepressants is a problem, why not just stay on them for the rest of one's life? Tardive dyskinesia is the quintessential example in which oppositional tolerance can produce withdrawal-like effects even while the patient keeps taking the medication. For antidepressants, oppositional tolerance would predict relapse into depression despite maintenance on antidepressants, sometimes referred to as antidepressant tachyphylaxis; this indeed occurs frequently (Kinrys et al., 2019). How much any given relapse is due to oppositional tolerance versus other factors is usually impossible to decide. Kinrys et al. (2019) state, "Tachyphylaxis may lead to TRD [treatment resistant depression], perhaps through a form of neuroreceptor tolerance or down-regulation."

The Internet forum on antidepressants and withdrawal from them, mentioned above, is called survivingantidepressants.org. The founder and moderator of that site reports communicating over a number of years with over 10,000 people who wanted support in withdrawing. The site contains many first-person accounts of withdrawal symptoms, which were in many cases very persistent. A recurring theme is that patients turn to peer support because of dismissive or otherwise unhelpful responses from prescribers. The site founder's narration of her own lived experience, as well as her review of literature on antidepressant withdrawal (Framer, 2021), is highly recommended reading.

Let's conclude the section on antidepressants, first with a statement by Fava, who as early as 2003 cited 136 studies suggesting a possible "Yes" answer to the question, "Can long-term treatment with antidepressant drugs worsen the course of depression?" Fava stated: "When drug treatment ends, oppositional processes may operate for some time, resulting in appearance of withdrawal symptoms and increased vulnerability to relapse. As Baldessarini remarks, the assumption that such physiological processes will readjust after a withdrawal phase is not supported by current awareness in the field of drug dependence" (p. 127). And according to Fava and Cosci (2019):

> A hidden conceptual assumption of a large body of research on treatment in depression is that … the receptor changes that are induced by antidepressants are limited to their time of administration or shortly afterward and that it is just a matter of allowing time for adaptation of the system to antidepressant discontinuation. This naive assumption runs counter to current concepts on the plasticity of the brain. The literature that we surveyed and, in particular, the oppositional model of tolerance, suggest that remission and recovery in mood disorders are a one-way street, characterized by structural remodeling of neural architecture and continually changing patterns of gene expression mediated by epigenetic mechanisms.

It is chilling to ponder the idea that the first-line drugs for anxiety, depression, obsessive-compulsive disorder, and premenstrual dysphoric disorder, while helping somewhat in the short run, may actually be harmful regarding the overall course, and that after decades of use and millions of long-term users, definitive answers on long-term effects are elusive. More chilling is Fava's (2003) suggestion that many may not want to see this question answered: "Certainly, researchers along these lines are likely to encounter tremendous difficulties in disclosing their results in journals or symposia or in getting their studies started and funded, in view of the current ideological and pharmaceutically driven climate. They should be ready to bear with the retaliation that outliers receive in these situations" (p. 130). That perspective remained unchanged 21 years later: Fava (2024) remarked, "The iatrogenic perspective is more than just ignored: it is forbidden" (p. 228).

4.6 Antipsychotics

In the mid-twentieth century, the antipsychotic drugs proved efficacious for psychosis (with chlorpromazine marketed in the USA in 1954), but gradually the withdrawal effects of tardive dyskinesia upon the motor system began to accumulate (see Paulson, 2005 for a narrative on the history of recognition of tardive dyskinesia, including clinicians' resistance to acknowledging it as a prevalent iatrogenic complication). Silvestri et al. (2000) found that people with antipsychotic treatment and withdrawal had increased sensitivity of D2 dopamine receptors. Moreover, patients with the highest upregulation of these receptors developed more severe tardive dyskinesia. The notion of tardive dyskinesia as a withdrawal problem related to dopaminergic transmission (with sometimes permanent effects) led to the idea, starting about 1978, that withdrawal of dopamine D2 receptor blockade could produce supersensitivity psychosis (see Chouinard et al., 2017, which includes a historical discussion of supersensitivity psychosis).

Read (2022) collected a sample of 585 people who had been on antipsychotics and tried to withdraw. "72% reported classical withdrawal effects of the kind associated with other central nervous system medications, including nausea, tremors, anxiety, agitation and headaches. 52% of these categorized those effects as 'severe'. 26% had tried four or more times to discontinue, and 23% took at least one year to successfully withdraw completely. In response to the open question, 73% reported one or more withdrawal effects, most frequently, insomnia, nervousness and extreme feelings; 26% reported one or more positive outcomes, most frequently more energy/alive and clearer thinking; and 18% reported psychosis" (p. 1).

In three of the cases with withdrawal psychosis, "there had been no primary or secondary diagnosis indicative of psychosis" (p. 4).

The notion that withdrawal from antipsychotic drugs can induce psychosis in people who were not psychotic in the first place is concerning, but an unsurprising corollary of the phenomenon of oppositional tolerance. Chouinard et al. (2017) reviewed the concept of dopamine supersensitivity psychosis resulting from antipsychotic drug treatment. They wrote:

"Davis and Rosenberg considered SP as a limbic equivalent of TD" (p. 190). "Data from animal studies show that chronic exposure to antipsychotic medications increases D2 receptor numbers most prominently in the caudate-putamen and the nucleus accumbens. Antipsychotic-induced dopamine supersensitivity is also linked to increased levels of D2 High receptors in these same brain regions" (p. 191).

4.7 Benzodiazepines

The benzodiazepines enjoyed huge popularity for anxiety, but the gradual accrual of evidence for tolerance and withdrawal effects dampened enthusiasm and produced cautionary guidelines (for history of benzodiazepines, see Wick, 2013). We mentioned earlier the downregulation of GABA transmission that results from treatment with benzodiazepines. The withdrawal syndrome from benzodiazepines can include anxiety, insomnia, rage, nightmares, intrusive thoughts, irritability, headache, depression, and, particularly for withdrawal from high doses, seizures and psychotic reactions (Onyett, 1989; Popish & Wells, 2025; Pétursson, 1994). Rickels et al. (1986) reported that over 75% of patients withdrawn from long-term use of benzodiazepines developed withdrawal symptoms. Nonetheless, the short-term efficacy of the benzodiazepines for anxiety (and possible long-term efficacy in some people) makes a large market for these drugs continue. Alprazolam was in the top 10 most prescribed psychotropic drugs, and 37th most widely prescribed of all drugs, as of 2023 (ClinCalc, 2025).

4.8 Sleeping Pills (Hypnotics)

The withdrawal effects, and recommendations for switching or deprescribing, for various sleeping pills have been reviewed by Watson et al. (2023). The results are not simple to summarize, since we are dealing with a very heterogeneous set. For benzodiazepines, the withdrawal effects are as above. For the z-drugs, zolpidem, zaleplon, and eszopiclone, when taken as directed, withdrawal problems are not much of a problem, probably because these drugs are of such short half-life that withdrawal takes place every day rather than having the intensity of withdrawal build up over time. For the DORA drugs, or dual orexin antagonists, serious withdrawal effects have not been proven so far, although a few cases have been reported that suggest such symptoms (Watson et al., 2023).

Antihistamines such as diphenhydramine and hydroxyzine have been used for sleep, and withdrawal symptoms of intense itching, hives, nasal congestion, insomnia, anxiety, headaches, and nausea have been reported—in other words, symptoms that are pretty much the opposite of the beneficial effects of the drugs (Myacare, 2025).

Melatonin, the sleep-rhythm-regulating hormone that is now sold over the counter in huge quantities and used as a sleeping pill, is one where there are still insufficient published studies for a conclusion. But there is reason to worry that years of exogenous melatonin, especially in the supra-physiological doses given in most marketed pills, may shut down the production of endogenous melatonin, and the mechanisms for endogenous production may atrophy from disuse. Or by other mechanisms, receptors may become less sensitive to endogenous melatonin. Interviews of sleep researchers Richard Wurtman, who played a large role in the discovery of the function of melatonin, and Michael Grandner, sleep researcher at the University of Pennsylvania, reflect these worries (Winkles, 2017). "According to Dr. Wurtman, melatonin supplements may work at first, but soon 'you'll stop responding because you desensitize the brain. And as a consequence, not only won't you respond to the stuff you take…you won't respond to the stuff you make, so it can actually promote insomnia after a period of time'" (p. 7). According to Michael Grandner, "Taking melatonin for an extended period of time, your body may acclimate and re-adjust and produce less over time which will work against you" (p. 8).

4.9 Migraine Headache Remedies

Mental health professionals (except for some biofeedback specialists and a few others) typically are not in the business of treating headaches. What do headaches have to do with mental health? Plenty! Migraine is reported to increase the risk for depression (by a factor of 2.5 according to Viudez-Martínez et al. (2024)), and the causal relationship is thought to be bidirectional. For migraine headaches, the triptans were ushered in with enthusiasm because of their efficacy in stopping short the progression of a headache. But gradually the evidence for withdrawal effects accumulated, and now it is well known that the number one cause of headaches becoming chronic is “medication overuse.” Medication overuse headache (MOH) can result from use of triptans, as well as ergots, NSAIDs, or opioids (Deighton et al., 2021). These authors state, “There is a need for migraine-specific medication that does not carry a risk of MOH.” This sentiment may be generalized to many other drugs acting upon the nervous system.

4.10 Other Drugs

The following is an incomplete list of drugs for which there is evidence of oppositional tolerance and/or withdrawal effects. References are supplied only for those not discussed elsewhere in the text. The finding of evidence for oppositional tolerance does not imply that the drug should not be given, of course. But this list is supplied to make the point that at least some oppositional tolerance and withdrawal effects, especially with drugs that affect neurons, are the rule rather than the exception:

1. Alcohol
2. Opiates
3. Barbiturates and other sedatives (Liappas et al., 1987)
4. Benzodiazepines
5. Cannabis (Kesner & Lovinger, 2021)
6. Anticonvulsants (Cosci & Chouinard, 2020)
7. Antipsychotics
8. Alpha 2 agonists (Reid et al., 1984)
9. Stimulants (Cosci & Chouinard, 2020)
10. Caffeine (Edwards et al., 2024)
11. Ketamine (Roxas et al., 2021)
12. Ergotamine
13. NSAIDs
14. Triptans
15. Tricyclics (Garner et al., 1993)
16. SSRIs and SNRIs
17. Beta blockers (Anık, 2022)
18. Nasal decongestants (Black & Remsen, 1980)
19. Proton pump inhibitors (Namikawa & Björnsson, 2024)
20. Antihistamines
21. Anticholinergics (McInnis & Petursson, 1984)
22. Insulin (Lewis et al., 2023)
23. Coenzyme Q 10 (Kalenikova et al., 2010)

When neuronal systems undergo oppositional tolerance, how permanent or long-lasting are the effects? If oppositional tolerance can be undone by withdrawing drugs "gradually" over a couple of weeks or a month, then it isn't much of a problem. On the other hand, if the homeostatic changes persist over long periods of time or are permanent, then the drugs can actually worsen the problems they were meant to solve.

The lesson that withdrawal effects can be permanent was taught to us convincingly by observations of tardive dyskinesia resulting from the antipsychotics. Although some dyskinesias do come and eventually disappear upon withdrawal of antipsychotics (and are deemed "withdrawal dyskinesias"), many do not ever disappear. Why are the changes for some people reversible and for others irreversible? The answer to this is unknown, at least to us.

4.11 Can Medicines Make Up for Problems with Learning and the Environment?

In the section of this book on psychoeducation, we will argue that mental health (as defined by the capacity to bring about happiness in oneself and others) is a complex set of learnable skills that interact with one another. For example, anger control, social interaction, conflict-resolution, self-discipline, kindness, decision-making, choice of self-talk, relaxation, and emotional regulation are all learned. Most often, through human history, these skills have been acquired through incidental learning rather than formal teaching: for example, the examples one sees in others, the rewards and punishments that life provides for various patterns, the value systems the culture imparts, and others. But they are also subject to deliberate training, as demonstrated by research on psychotherapy and psychoeducation. If we imagine a pill that imparts those skills, circumventing the necessity for learning experiences, we should also imagine that pills will produce virtuosity in piano playing, dancing, chess, basketball shooting, writing, mathematics, and other skills. Such a vision is implausible. In the meantime, we already have learning-based procedures that tend to increase proficiency in all of the skills listed above, and others.

Similar reasoning applies to environmental influences, and the implausibility that drugs can supersede these. For example, a woman comes to treatment for depression. She has moved to a town where she has no social network, to take care of elderly parents who have now died; she works in a tedious job with an abusive supervisor, to make financial ends meet, and she has little time or opportunity for making friends. It is implausible that taking a pill would render her happy, without some change in her environment. It may be argued that medication might give her the energy to change her environment. But there are many environmental circumstances that people find themselves unable to change.

4.12 Final Thoughts on the Possibility of Long-Term Harm

You are not likely to find the ideas of this chapter in most "mainstream" textbooks of psychiatry or psychopharmacology. But the more we look, the more impressive the accumulation of evidence for the problems of oppositional tolerance becomes. If it turns out that important psychotropic drugs help in the short run but do harm in the long run, that would not be the first time that short- and long-term effects turn out to be in conflict with one another. And, with randomized trials viewed as the gold standard of proof, and near-impossibility of conducting randomized trials to assess the very long-term effects of psychotropic drugs, it is not surprising that after all these years, we are still uncertain about long-term effects. Although uncertainty still remains, evidence to date is sufficient to recommend that if there are learning-based methods and pharmacological methods available which both appear efficacious for a condition, the learning-based approaches, all other things equal, are less likely to have iatrogenic consequences. And when medications such as the antidepressants, the antipsychotics (particularly when used for conditions other than psychosis), or the benzodiazepines are employed, usually there should be strong efforts to employ learning-based methods to permit discontinuation as soon as possible, before oppositional tolerance has had a long time to proceed. This recommendation is quite different from current practice, where these medications are frequently the only treatment, and are continued indefinitely.

We're aware that many patients are simply unwilling or unable to participate in learning-based treatment, and that at times even the best learning-based treatment doesn't act fast enough. We're aware that many times suffering is so great that the short-term consequences of withholding medication outweigh the long-term dependency issues we worry about. If our primary purpose were to advise medical personnel, we would advise *oppositional-tolerance-informed* decision-making, both for providers and for patients—to take the phenomenon into account with every medication decision, and to weigh it and other potential risks against the predicted benefits.

But our primary purpose is not to give pharmacological advice, but to elucidate the limitations of the biomedical model as a way of improving the mental health of society. The strategy of screening more people, providing more medications to a higher fraction of people, and persuading people not to go off medication, while hoping for future pharmacologic breakthroughs, is really the primary mental health strategy some would advocate. The evidence reviewed in this chapter makes us skeptical that this strategy will relieve the societal burden of psychopathology.

References

Andrews, P. W., Kornstein, S. G., Halberstadt, L. J., Gardner, C. O., & Neale, M. C. (2011). Blue again: Perturbational effects of antidepressants suggest monoaminergic homeostasis in major depression. *Frontiers in Psychology, 2*, 159. https://doi.org/10.3389/fpsyg.2011.00159

Anık, A. (2022). Beta-blocker rebound phenomenon in an adolescent with graves' disease. *Journal of Clinical Research in Pediatric Endocrinology, 14*(4), 490–491. https://doi.org/10.4274/jcrpe.galenos.2022.2022-6-2

Barbosa Eyler, G. E. (2023). ¿Apatía o embotamiento emocional por ISRS? Una revisión de la literatura. *Vertex (Buenos Aires, Argentina), 34*(161, Jul.-Sept.), 61–66. https://doi.org/10.53680/vertex.v34i161.486

Black, M. J., & Remsen, K. A. (1980) Rhinitis medicamentosa. *Canadian Medical Association Journal, 122*(8), 881–884.

Brody, D. J., & Gu, Q. (2020). *Antidepressant use among adults: United States, 2015–2018*. National Center for Health Statistics. (Data Brief No. 377). https://www.cdc.gov/nchs/products/databriefs/db377.htm

Castellanos, F. X., Lee, P. P., Sharp, W., Jeffries, N. O., Greenstein, D. K., Clasen, L. S., Blumenthal, J. D., James, R. S., Ebens, C. L., Walter, J. M., Zijdenbos, A., Evans, A. C., Giedd, J. N., & Rapoport, J. L. (2002). Developmental trajectories of brain volume abnormalities in children and adolescents with attention-deficit/hyperactivity disorder. *JAMA, 288*(14), 1740–1748.

Catalan, A., Salazar de Pablo, G., Aymerich, C., Guinart, D., Goena, J., Madaria, L., Pacho, M., Alameda, L., Garrido-Torres, N., Pedruzo, B., Rubio, J. M., Gonzalez-Torres, M. A., Fusar-Poli, P., & Correll, C. U. (2025). "Short" versus "long" duration of untreated psychosis in people with first-episode psychosis: A systematic review and meta-analysis of baseline status and follow-up outcomes. *Schizophrenia Bulletin, 51*(5), 1206–1230. https://doi.org/10.1093/schbul/sbae201

Chouinard, G., Samaha, A. N., Chouinard, V. A., Peretti, C. S., Kanahara, N., Takase, M., & Iyo, M. (2017). Antipsychotic-induced dopamine Supersensitivity psychosis: Pharmacology, criteria, and therapy. *Psychotherapy and Psychosomatics, 86*(4), 189–219. https://doi.org/10.1159/000477313

Cipriani, A., Zhou, X., Del Giovane, C., Hetrick, S. E., Qin, B., Whittington, C., Coghill, D., Zhang, Y., Hazell, P., Leucht, S., Cuijpers, P., Pu, J., Cohen, D., Ravindran, A. V., Liu, Y., Michael, K. D., Yang, L., Liu, L., & Xie, P. (2016). Comparative efficacy and tolerability of antidepressants for major depressive disorder in children and adolescents: A network meta-analysis. *Lancet, 388*(10047), 881–890. https://doi.org/10.1016/S0140-6736(16)30385-3

Clincalc. (2025). *The top 300 of 2023: ClinCalc DrugStats database*. https://clincalc.com/DrugStats/Top300Drugs.aspx

Cohen, L. S., Altshuler, L. L., Harlow, B. L., Nonacs, R., Newport, D. J., Viguera, A. C., Suri, R., Burt, V. K., Hendrick, V., Reminick, A. M., Loughead, A., Vitonis, A. F., & Stowe, Z. N. (2006). Relapse of major depression during pregnancy in women who maintain or discontinue antidepressant treatment. *JAMA, 295*(5), 499–507. https://doi.org/10.1001/jama.295.5.499

Coleman, K. J. (2013). Use of antipsychotic medications in pediatric populations: What do the data say? *Current Psychiatry Reports, 15*(12), 426. https://doi.org/10.1007/s11920-013-0426-8. (Erratum published 2014: Current Psychiatry Reports, 16(2), 432.).

Cosci, F., & Chouinard, G. (2020). Acute and persistent withdrawal syndromes following discontinuation of psychotropic medications. *Psychotherapy and Psychosomatics, 89*(5), 283–306. https://doi.org/10.1159/000506868

Cosci, F., & Fava, G. A. (2021). Prescribing pharmacotherapy for major depressive disorder: How does a clinician decide? *Biomedicine Hub, 6*(3), 118–121. https://doi.org/10.1159/000519656

Deighton, A. M., Harris, L. A., Johnston, K., et al. (2021). The burden of medication overuse headache and patterns of switching and discontinuation among triptan users: A systematic literature review. *BMC Neurology, 21*, 425. https://doi.org/10.1186/s12883-021-02451-x

Dennis, J. A., Gittner, L. S., Payne, J. D., & Nugent, K. (2020). Characteristics of U.S. adults taking prescription antipsychotic medications: National Health and nutrition examination survey 2013–2018. *BMC Psychiatry, 20*(1), 483. https://doi.org/10.1186/s12888-020-02895-4

Dharavath, R. N., Pina-Leblanc, C., Tang, V. M., Sloan, M. E., Nikolova, Y. S., Pangarov, P., Ruocco, A. C., Shield, K., Voineskos, D., Blumberger, D. M., Boileau, I., Bozinoff, N., Gerretsen, P., Vieira, E., Melamed, O. C., Sibille, E., Quilty, L. C., & Prevot, T. D. (2023). GABAergic signaling in alcohol use disorder and withdrawal: Pathological involvement and therapeutic potential. *Frontiers in Neural Circuits, 17*, 1218737. https://doi.org/10.3389/fncir.2023.1218737

Edwards, F., Bright, M., Dux, C., Coyer, F., & Laupland, K. B. (2024). Caffeine consumption and withdrawal among patients in the intensive care unit. *Australian Critical Care, 37*(3), 436–440. https://doi.org/10.1016/j.aucc.2023.03.004

Fava, G. A. (2003). Can long-term treatment with antidepressant drugs worsen the course of depression? *Journal of Clinical Psychiatry, 64*(2), 123–133. https://doi.org/10.4088/jcp.v64n0204

Fava, G. A. (2020). May antidepressant drugs worsen the conditions they are supposed to treat? The clinical foundations of the oppositional model of tolerance. *Therapeutic Advances in Psychopharmacology, 10*, 2045125320970325. https://doi.org/10.1177/2045125320970325

Fava, G. A. (2024). The clinical meaning of withdrawal with antidepressant drugs. *Psychotherapy and Psychosomatics, 93*(4), 224–229. https://doi.org/10.1159/000540033

Fava, G. A., & Cosci, F. (2019). Understanding and managing withdrawal syndromes after discontinuation of antidepressant drugs. *Journal of Clinical Psychiatry, 80*(6), 19com12794. https://doi.org/10.4088/JCP.19com12794

Framer, A. (2021). What I have learnt from helping thousands of people taper off antidepressants and other psychotropic medications. *Therapeutic Advances in Psychopharmacology, 11*, 2045125321991274. https://doi.org/10.1177/2045125321991274

Garland, E. L., Froeliger, B., Zeidan, F., Partin, K., & Howard, M. O. (2013). The downward spiral of chronic pain, prescription opioid misuse, and addiction: Cognitive, affective, and neuropsychopharmacologic pathways. *Neuroscience and Biobehavioral Reviews, 37*(10 Pt 2), 2597–2607. https://doi.org/10.1016/j.neubiorev.2013.08.006

Garner, E. M., Kelly, M. W., & Thompson, D. F. (1993). Tricyclic antidepressant withdrawal syndrome. *Annals of Pharmacotherapy, 27*(9), 1068–1072. https://doi.org/10.1177/106002809302700912

Glasziou, P., Chalmers, I., Rawlins, M., & McCulloch, P. (2007). When are randomised trials unnecessary? Picking signal from noise. *BMJ, 334*(7589), 349–351. https://doi.org/10.1136/bmj.39070.527986.68

Glenmullen, J. (2000). *Prozac backlash: Overcoming the dangers of Prozac, Zoloft, Paxil, and other antidepressants with safe, effective alternatives*. Simon & Schuster.

Hengartner, M. P., & Plöderl, M. (2022). Estimates of the minimal important difference to evaluate the clinical significance of antidepressants in the acute treatment of moderate-to-severe depression. *BMJ Evidence-Based Medicine, 27*(2), 69–73. https://doi.org/10.1136/bmjebm-2020-111600

Henssler, J., Schmidt, Y., Schmidt, U., Schwarzer, G., Bschor, T., & Baethge, C. (2024). Incidence of antidepressant discontinuation symptoms: A systematic review and meta-analysis. *Lancet Psychiatry, 11*(7), 526–535. https://doi.org/10.1016/S2215-0366(24)00133-0

Hieronymus, F., Jauhar, S., Østergaard, S. D., & Young, A. H. (2020). One (effect) size does not fit at all: Interpreting clinical significance and effect sizes in depression treatment trials. *Journal of Psychopharmacology, 34*(10), 1074–1078. https://doi.org/10.1177/0269881120922950

Jakobsen, J. C., Katakam, K. K., Schou, A., Hellmuth, S. G., Stallknecht, S. E., Leth-Møller, K., Iversen, M., Banke, M. B., Petersen, I. J., Klingenberg, S. L., Krogh, J., Ebert, S. E., Timm, A., Lindschou, J., & Gluud, C. (2017). Selective serotonin reuptake inhibitors versus placebo in patients with major depressive disorder. A systematic review with meta-analysis and Trial sequential analysis. *BMC Psychiatry, 17*(1), 58. https://doi.org/10.1186/s12888-016-1173-2

Jakubovski, E., Johnson, J. A., Nasir, M., Müller-Vahl, K., & Bloch, M. H. (2019). Systematic review and meta-analysis: Dose-response curve of SSRIs and SNRIs in anxiety disorders. *Depression and Anxiety, 36*(3), 198–212. https://doi.org/10.1002/da.22854

Kalenikova, E., Gorodetskay, E., Konovalova, E., Medvedev, O., Ruuge, E., and Lankin, V. (2010). Coenzyme Q10 long-term supplementation may result in withdrawal effect in myocardium: PP. 13.492 *Journal of Hypertension, 28*, e198-e199, 2010. https://doi.org/10.1097/01.hjh.0000378817.00584.b1

Kesner, A. J., & Lovinger, D. M. (2021). Cannabis use, abuse, and withdrawal: Cannabinergic mechanisms, clinical, and preclinical findings. *Journal of Neurochemistry, 157*(5), 1674–1696. https://doi.org/10.1111/jnc.15369

Kinrys, G., Gold, A. K., Pisano, V. D., Freeman, M. P., Papakostas, G. I., Mischoulon, D., Nierenberg, A. A., & Fava, M. (2019). Tachyphylaxis in major depressive disorder: A review of the current state of research. *Journal of Affective Disorders, 245*, 488–497. https://doi.org/10.1016/j.jad.2018.10.357

Lewis, S. T., Greenway, F., Tucker, T. R., Alexander, M., Jackson, L. K., Hepford, S. A., Loveridge, B., & Lakey, J. R. T. (2023). A receptor story: Insulin resistance pathophysiology and physiologic insulin resensitization's role as a treatment modality. *International Journal of Molecular Sciences, 24*(13), 10927. https://doi.org/10.3390/ijms241310927

Liappas, I. A., Jenner, F. A., & Vicente, B. (1987). Withdrawal syndromes. *Journal of the Royal College of Physicians of London, 21*(3), 214–218.

Masdrakis, V. G., Markianos, M., & Baldwin, D. S. (2023). Apathy associated with antidepressant drugs: A systematic review. *Acta Neuropsychiatrica, 35*(4), 189–204. https://doi.org/10.1017/neu.2023.6

McCabe, C., Mishor, Z., Cowen, P. J., & Harmer, C. J. (2010). Diminished neural processing of aversive and rewarding stimuli during selective serotonin reuptake inhibitor treatment. *Biological Psychiatry, 67*(5), 439–445. https://doi.org/10.1016/j.biopsych.2009.11.001

McInnis, M., & Petursson, H. (1984). Trihexyphenidyl dependence. *Acta Psychiatrica Scandinavica, 69*(6), 538–542. https://doi.org/10.1111/j.1600-0447.1984.tb02528.x

Moncrieff, J., Hobday, H., Sørensen, A., Read, J., Plöderl, M., Hengartner, M., Kamp, C., Jakobsen, J., Juul, S., Davies, J., & Horowitz, M. (2025). Evidence on antidepressant withdrawal: An appraisal and reanalysis of a recent systematic review. *Psychological Medicine, 55*, e191. https://doi.org/10.1017/S0033291725100652

Myacare. (2025). *Antihistamine withdrawal: Dependence, withdrawal symptoms, management and more*. https://myacare.com/blog/antihistamine-withdrawal-dependence-withdrawal-symptoms-management-and-more

Nader, M. A., Morgan, D., Gage, H. D., Nader, S. H., Calhoun, T. L., Buchheimer, N., Ehrenkaufer, R., & Mach, R. H. (2006). PET imaging of dopamine D2 receptors during chronic cocaine self-administration in monkeys. *Nature Neuroscience, 9*(8), 1050–1056. https://doi.org/10.1038/nn1737

Namikawa, K., & Björnsson, E. S. (2024). Rebound acid hypersecretion after withdrawal of long-term proton pump inhibitor (ppi) treatment-are ppis addictive? *International Journal of Molecular Sciences, 25*(10), 5459. https://doi.org/10.3390/ijms25105459

Nicotra, C. M., & Strawn, J. R. (2023). Advances in pharmacotherapy for pediatric anxiety disorders. *Child and Adolescent Psychiatric Clinics of North America, 32*(3), 573–587. https://doi.org/10.1016/j.chc.2023.02.006

Onyett, S. R. (1989). The benzodiazepine withdrawal syndrome and its management. *Journal of the Royal College of General Practitioners, 39*(321), 160–163.

Papp, A., & Onton, J. A. (2022). Triggers and characteristics of brain zaps according to the findings of an Internet questionnaire. *The Primary Care Companion for CNS Disorders, 24*(1), https://doi.org/10.4088/PCC.21m02972

Paulson, G. W. (2005). Historical comments on tardive dyskinesia: A neurologist's perspective. *Journal of Clinical Psychiatry, 66*(2), 260–264. https://doi.org/10.4088/jcp.v66n0216

Peleg, L. C., Rabinovitch, D., Lavie, Y., Rabbie, D. M., Horowitz, I., Fruchter, E., & Gruenwald, I. (2022). Post-SSRI sexual dysfunction (PSSD): Biological plausibility, symptoms, diagnosis, and presumed risk factors. *Sexual Medicine Reviews, 10*(1), 91–98. https://doi.org/10.1016/j.sxmr.2021.07.001

Pétursson, H. (1994). The benzodiazepine withdrawal syndrome. *Addiction, 89*(11), 1455–1459. https://doi.org/10.1111/j.1360-0443.1994.tb03743.x

Popish, S. J., & Wells, D. L. (2025). *Re-evaluating the use of benzodiazepines: A focus on high-risk populations*. U.S. Department of Veterans Affairs, Pharmacy Benefits Management Academic Detailing Service. https://downloads.asam.org/sitefinity-production-blobs/docs/default-source/guidelines/benzodiazepine-tapering-2025/va_high-risk-populations.pdf

Pratt, L. A., Brody, D. J., & Gu, Q. (2017). Antidepressant use among persons aged 12 and over: United States, 2011–2014. *NCHS Data Brief*, No. 283. https://www.cdc.gov/nchs/data/databriefs/db283.pdf

Price, J., Cole, V., & Goodwin, G. M. (2009). Emotional side effects of selective serotonin reuptake inhibitors: Qualitative study. *British Journal of Psychiatry, 195*, 211–217.

Read, J. (2020). How common and severe are six withdrawal effects from, and addiction to, antidepressants? The experiences of a large international sample of patients. *Addictive Behaviors, 102*, 106157. https://doi.org/10.1016/j.addbeh.2019.106157

Read, J. (2022). The experiences of 585 people when they tried to withdraw from antipsychotic drugs. *Addictive Behaviors Reports, 15*, 100421. https://doi.org/10.1016/j.abrep.2022.100421

Reid, J. L., Campbell, B. C., & Hamilton, C. A. (1984). Withdrawal reactions following cessation of central alpha-adrenergic receptor agonists. *Hypertension, 6*(5 Pt 2), II71–II75. https://doi.org/10.1161/01.hyp.6.5_pt_2.ii71

Reports and Data. (2025). *Market report: Hypnotics and sedatives market*. https://www.reportsanddata.com/report-detail/hypnotics-and-sedatives-market

Rickels, K., Case, W. G., Schweizer, E. E., Swenson, C., & Fridman, R. B. (1986). Low-dose dependence in chronic benzodiazepine users: A preliminary report on 119 patients. *Psychopharmacology Bulletin, 22*(2), 407–415.

Roxas, N., Ahuja, C., Isom, J., Wilkinson, S. T., & Capurso, N. (2021). A potential case of acute ketamine withdrawal: Clinical implications for the treatment of refractory depression. *American Journal of Psychiatry, 178*(7), 588–591. https://doi.org/10.1176/appi.ajp.2020.20101480

Sansone, R. A., & Sansone, L. A. (2010). SSRI-induced indifference. *Psychiatry, 7*(10), 14–18.

Shaw, P., Sharp, W. S., Morrison, M., Eckstrand, K., Greenstein, D. K., Clasen, L. S., Evans, A. C., & Rapoport, J. L. (2009). Psychostimulant treatment and the developing cortex in attention deficit hyperactivity disorder. *American Journal of Psychiatry, 166*(1), 58–63. https://doi.org/10.1176/appi.ajp.2008.08050781

Silvestri, S., Seeman, M. V., Negrete, J. C., Houle, S., Shammi, C. M., Remington, G. J., Kapur, S., Zipursky, R. B., Wilson, A. A., Christensen, B. K., & Seeman, P. (2000). Increased dopamine D2 receptor binding after long-term treatment with antipsychotics in humans: A clinical PET study. *Psychopharmacology, 152*(2), 174–180. https://doi.org/10.1007/s002130000532

Slee, A., Nazareth, I., Bondaronek, P., Liu, Y., Cheng, Z., & Freemantle, N. (2019). Pharmacological treatments for generalised anxiety disorder: A systematic review and network meta-analysis. *Lancet, 393*(10173), 768–777. https://doi.org/10.1016/S0140-6736(18)31793-8

Smith, G. C. S., & Pell, J. P. (2003). Parachute use to prevent death and major trauma related to gravitational challenge: Systematic review of randomised controlled trials. *BMJ, 327*, 1459–1461. https://doi.org/10.1136/bmj.327.7429.1459

Strayhorn, J. M. (2021). Virtual controls as an alternative to randomized controlled trials for assessing efficacy of interventions. *BMC Medical Research Methodology, 21*, 3. https://doi.org/10.1186/s12874-020-01191-9

Strayhorn, J. M. (2026). Disorders with irritability, aggression, etc. in official criteria. https://josephstrayhornmd.com/speeches/dsm_disorders_and_aggression.pdf

van der Pal, Z., Walhovd, K. B., Amlien, I. K., Guichelaar, C. J., Kaiser, A., Bottelier, M. A., Geurts, H. M., Reneman, L., & Schrantee, A. (2024). Stimulant medication use and apparent cortical thickness development in attention-deficit/hyperactivity disorder: A prospective longitudinal study. *Frontiers in Psychiatry, 15*, 1365159. https://doi.org/10.3389/fpsyt.2024.1365159

Viudez-Martínez, A., Torregrosa, A. B., Navarrete, F., & García-Gutiérrez, M. S. (2024). Understanding the biological relationship between migraine and depression. *Biomolecules, 14*(2), 163. https://doi.org/10.3390/biom14020163

Volkow, N. D., Fowler, J. S., Wang, G.-J., Hitzemann, R., Logan, J., Schlyer, D., Dewey, S. L., & Wolf, A. P. (1993). Decreased dopamine D2 receptor availability is associated with reduced frontal metabolism in cocaine abusers. *Synapse, 14*(2), 169–177.

Walhovd, K. B., Amlien, I., Schrantee, A., Rohani, D. A., Groote, I., Bjørnerud, A., Fjell, A. M., & Reneman, L. (2020). Methylphenidate effects on cortical thickness in children and adults with attention-deficit/hyperactivity disorder: A randomized clinical trial. *American Journal of Neuroradiology, 41*(5), 758–765. https://doi.org/10.3174/ajnr.A6560

Warlick, H. G., De Souza, G. N., & Gallicchio, V. S. (2020). Restoration of GABA-a receptor function after benzodiazepine use: A meta-analysis. *Journal of Stem Cell Research, 1*(1), 1–19. Accessed Feb 11, 2026, from https://www.researchgate.net/publication/351521646_Restoration_Of_GABAA_Receptor_Function_After_Benzodiazepine_Use_A_Meta-Analysis

Watson, N. F., Benca, R. M., Krystal, A. D., McCall, W. V., & Neubauer, D. N. (2023). Alliance for sleep clinical practice guideline on switching or deprescribing hypnotic medications for insomnia. *Journal of Clinical Medicine, 12*(7), 2493. https://doi.org/10.3390/jcm12072493

Wick, J. Y. (2013). The history of benzodiazepines. *The Consultant Pharmacist., 28*(9), 538–548. https://doi.org/10.4140/TCP.n.2013.538

Winkles, V. (2017). *The dark side of melatonin.* https://www.huffpost.com/entry/the-dark-side-of-melatoni_b_8855998.

Wyatt, R. J. (1991). Neuroleptics and the natural course of schizophrenia. *Schizophrenia Bulletin, 17*(2), 325–351. https://doi.org/10.1093/schbul/17.2.325

Chapter 5
Can Psychotherapy Relieve the Societal Burden of Psychopathology?

Abstract From Freudian origins where free association was the agenda of most sessions, psychotherapy has moved toward more use of educational methods, as for example in cognitive behavior therapy. Manuals, curricula, workbooks, and homework assignments (a.k.a. action plans) are common. And the evidence for the efficacy of psychotherapies for a variety of conditions has been established without question, although such evidence usually does not report large fractions of complete remissions or cures. When research studies "psychotherapy," it usually means around 12 to 20 h of contact. This number has been arrived at more to ensure timely completion of studies than to address adequately the number and complexity of the skills needed for psychological health. The times on task required by other skills, such as sports, music, mathematics, and language learning, lead to doubt that 12 to 20 h should be sacrosanct. But even if 12 to 20 h of contact were sufficient, research strongly suggests that only small fractions of the total population with a given condition obtain that much treatment. High utilizers of psychotherapy absorb a large fraction of the total professional labor. Given economic forces and current distributions of psychotherapeutic effort, psychotherapy cannot relieve the societal burden of psychopathology.

Keywords Psychotherapy · Time on task · Educational methods · Distributions · Barriers to treatment

Psychotherapy is in many ways a beautiful invention. Two (or more) people work in a cooperative venture to improve the mental health of at least one of them. The methods of science are employed to answer the question of how they should work together most effectively. The enterprise seems to work best in the presence of good relationships: those with mutual trust, empathy, honesty, warmth, good listening, rational thinking, and cooperative versus adversarial orientation.

Furthermore, the evidence tells us that psychotherapy can have life-changing positive effects. The efficacy for anxiety and depression has been very widely studied, especially for behavior therapy and cognitive behavior therapy (Beck, 2021).

J. M. Strayhorn, Jr. et al., *The Promise of Psychoeducation in Relieving the Societal Burden of Psychopathology*, SpringerBriefs in Modern Perspectives on Disability Research, https://doi.org/10.1007/978-981-92-0922-4_1

For anger control and aggression, the results have been compiled into at least 21 meta-analyses as of 2018 (Lee & DiGiuseppe, 2018). Psychotherapy has been found useful even for conditions that are quintessentially biological in nature: psychosis, including hallucinations (Chadwick, 2006; Craig et al., 2018), and bipolar disorder (Frank et al., 2005). Positive results are reported for children as well as adults. Parent training has repeatedly proved efficacious for various disorders in children, especially disruptive behavior (Kazdin, 2005); also some evidence supports its efficacy with other disorders, including children's anxiety (Lebowitz et al., 2020), obsessive-compulsive disorder (Lebowitz & Shimshoni, 2018), and avoidant-restrictive food intake disorder (Shimshoni et al., 2020).

In keeping with the idea of mental health as a set of learnable skills, psychotherapeutic techniques, especially those of behavior therapy, cognitive behavior therapy, dialectical behavior therapy, and parent training, have moved more and more toward an explicit skills learning orientation. Early behavior therapists used desensitization to teach emotional regulation, and social skills training and assertion skills training to help with interpersonal dealings (Wolpe, 1973). Dialectical behavior therapy focuses on skills of mindfulness, distress tolerance, emotional regulation, and interpersonal effectiveness (Linehan, 1993). Positive affect treatment (Craske et al., 2022) gives patients a different worksheet each week, to be filled out daily, in the service of skills of mobilizing pleasant emotions. Cognitive behavior therapy for depression relies heavily upon the skill of choosing one's own self-talk in ways that maximize quality of life.

Even psychodynamic therapy can be thought of as operating through learning of psychological skills, although the promotion of learning is much less didactic. Transference-oriented psychoanalytic therapy can be seen as emphasizing the important skill of discernment of other people's characters and motives, based on current evidence and not on distorted perceptions derived from past relationships. Psychoanalytic therapy aimed at making the unconscious conscious can be seen as promoting the skill of awareness of one's own emotions, motives, thoughts, wishes, and conflicts. Psychoanalytic therapy aimed at "separation-individuation" can be seen as promoting the skill of independent thinking and action. Indeed, if we define learning as change in behavior (including thought and emotion) as a result of experience, and if we define a skill as a pattern of behavior (including thought and emotion) that can be learned, all psychotherapy is by definition learning-based and skill-based.

The capacity of the human brain to alter itself through learning, particularly repetitive and hierarchically arranged practice, is nothing short of amazing. To observe the performances of not just virtuosos, but just respectably competent musicians, gymnasts, divers, jugglers, chess-players, magicians, dancers, and athletes in numerous other sports, gives an immediate visual confirmation that the brain can accomplish things that for the novice would be impossible. In each case, the brain has been altered by many hours of progressive practice. The same amazing transformation is visible in the world of difference between the respectably competent writer, speaker, mathematician, reader, or creator of scientific progress, on the one hand, and the novice or unschooled person in these areas on the other. Psychotherapy works its magic by harnessing the amazing power of learning.

The main idea of this chapter is that despite all the benefits of psychotherapy, when competently facilitated by the therapist and earnestly worked at by the patient, psychotherapy is unlikely to relieve the societal burden of psychopathology. Why? Because it is so difficult to deliver enough of it—to achieve enough time on task.

Most of the studies of psychotherapy have involved a fairly low amount of time on task in learning, at least if the time is measured by direct face-to-face time with the therapist. For example, a meta-analysis of therapeutic approaches to anger (Saini, 2009) reported a mean of 8.5 therapy sessions; the number of sessions was positively related to treatment effect. Various studies of cognitive therapy have established a de facto standard of around 12 to 20 sessions, of about an hour each. For example, a study by Bruijniks et al. (2020) specified a maximum of 20 sessions; Schnurr et al. (2007) used 10 90-min sessions. Flückiger et al. (2020) observed, "In randomized clinical trials, the number of sessions is typically fixed to deliver manualized treatments and to control for dosage effects (e.g., in a 16-session format)."

As such, it could be that the positive results from a few hours of psychotherapy represent the harvesting of low hanging fruit: perhaps studies tend to select the people who are skilled enough in most areas of life that a limited amount of work in a certain area is enough to result in positive functioning. And/or participants are recruited who are motivated enough to carry out assignments for practice of skills outside therapy sessions.

How much time does it take to learn all the skills of mental health, starting from scratch? Or how much time does it take to learn any one of them, given a very low skill level to begin with? The answer to this question is unknown. And any answer would probably be quite complex, with the amount of time required dependent on the person's past experience, their IQ, their motivation level, their skill levels in various other areas, and so forth. And even with all variables specified, the answer would probably be in the form of averages with large standard deviations.

We can get something of a feeling for how much time on task it takes for skill learning by looking at the number of hours required for various skills outside what's usually thought of as the psychological skill arena. Here are some estimates of the amount of time required to become expert in various skills:

Professional level violin: Around 10,000 h (Ericsson & Pool, 2016; Ericsson et al., 1993).

Becoming a concert pianist: About 1400 h a year during the teen years (Bloom, 1985).

Becoming a competitive amateur swimmer: 600 to 800 hours a year during the preteen years, 1250 to 1450 h a year during the teen years. (Bloom, 1985).

For an English speaker to learn Spanish well enough for a foreign service job: About 600 class hours (US Department of State, Foreign Service Institute, 2026).

For an English speaker to learn Mandarin or Japanese well enough for a foreign service job: About 2200 class hours (US Department of State, Foreign Service Institute, 2026).

Typical time spent in a K-12 school year, in USA: About 1230 h a year (Kraft & Novicoff, 2022).

State of New York, practice time required driving before taking road test: at least 50 h (New York State Department of Motor Vehicles, 2026).

Amount of work time estimated for a 3 credit hour college course: 135 h (Code of Federal Regulations, 2026).

Suppose we add to this list:

Amount of time for a chronically depressed, anxious, or aggressive person to learn, via psychotherapy, the skills that remedy these problems: between 12 and 20 face-to-face hours.

Does it seem that "One of these things is not like the others?"

If ordinary people are capable of investing more than a thousand hours into practice with a musical instrument or in a sport, and if we have millions of people sinking several thousand hours into work on competence in videogames, what's the problem with people's putting as much time as needed into work on emotional regulation, interpersonal relationship skills, development of good will, and other skills that are much more important for the quality of life?

Before we ask why they don't, let's first look at the evidence that indeed, on the average, they don't.

Strayhorn et al. (2025) accessed about 32,000 electronic medical records of people diagnosed with Intermittent Explosive Disorder, and computed the distribution of the number of psychotherapy sessions people obtained. Seventy-five percent received no psychotherapy. Only 10% attended 9 sessions or more. 7.5% attended 14 sessions or more, and only 2.5% attended 40 sessions or more. Lots of psychotherapeutic labor was expended, though—but it was devoted very disproportionately to the high utilizers. The 7.5% of patients who attended 14 sessions or more received 80% of the total psychotherapy hours. The 2.5% who attended 40 sessions or more received about half the total psychotherapeutic labor.

These numbers tend to make the case that psychotherapy will not make a big dent in the problem of impulsive aggression in society: only a small fraction of people with this problem, at least according to this database, received anywhere close to enough psychotherapy to make a difference. With this shape of distribution, doubling the psychotherapeutic labor pool would not change this.

Perhaps people with impulsive aggression are less tolerant of psychotherapy? To check the generality of our first finding, we then (Strayhorn & Zhang-James, in preparation) accessed about 3.7 million electronic medical records of people with diagnoses of Major Depressive Disorder. This time, the distribution of the psychotherapeutic labor was even more lopsided in the direction of the high utilizers, with even higher fractions of people receiving too little psychotherapy to make a difference. Again, so much of the psychotherapeutic labor is absorbed by the high utilizers, and there are so many who utilize in insignificant or zero amounts, that we should not count on psychotherapy to solve the societal problem of depression—assuming, of course, that the 3.7 million we accessed were a representative sample.

Other research has pointed to the predominance of pharmacological treatment over psychotherapy, including for children. Of 75,024 privately insured children getting medications prescribed for anxiety, 65% had received less than 2 sessions of psychotherapy before prescription (Bushnell et al., 2019). Of those without psychotherapy before, 70% received no psychotherapy after being prescribed medication. According to Hincapie-Castillo et al. (2017), of 24,372 Medicaid children getting prescriptions for antipsychotics, a little less than half had received a "psychosocial service" in the 3 months before initiation.

How can we account for these findings? Why do so few people get psychotherapy in the amount that would appear to be adequate time on task? Most psychotherapists tend to work during normal working hours, the same hours that most potential patients have to be at work or school. For a patient to be able to take off an hour from work, week after week, is likely an unusual circumstance, even if psychotherapy is delivered with zero travel time. If therapy is delivered by telehealth, there may not be a private place the patient can go during the time off work. If treatment is in person, much time may be required for travel, especially for rural residents and especially for those dependent upon buses or other public transportation. Then we have the cost of psychotherapy, which is a subset of health care costs. Often there are copays or deductibles that make even psychotherapy which is officially covered by insurance too costly. And if psychotherapy were delivered in adequate amounts to all the people whose diagnoses warrant it, the costs would almost certainly either bankrupt insurance companies or lead to a massive increase in premiums. The solvency of the insurance industry depends on the condition that most people who can use psychotherapy will not get it.

The mismatch between the numbers of people with mental health problems and the current systems for delivering psychotherapy to them led Kazdin and Blase (2011) to conclude, "The need for psychological services is enormous, and only a small proportion of individuals in need actually receive treatment. Individual psychotherapy, the dominant model of treatment delivery, is not likely to be able to meet this need" (p. 21). These authors called for the harnessing of Internet and smartphones, nonprofessionals, self-help groups, and the media in reducing the societal burden of psychopathology. As we will discuss, these are areas where psychoeducation is the frontier.

There is still stigma associated with obtaining mental health treatment, and perhaps elimination of such stigma would increase the impact of psychotherapy upon mental health. But it appears that the major limitation is that psychotherapy is part of the health care system, and not part of the educational system. Here are some of the characteristics of the provision of health care:

1. There is the presumption that most health care providers will spend, at most, a few hours a year with any given patient.
2. There is a presumption that aside from regular check-ups and preventive intervention such as vaccinations and dental cleanings, medical services are delivered only in case of illness—"medical necessity"—but not otherwise.

3. The medical insurance industry is based on the presumption that many people pay premiums, but few need more payments for services than the total amount of premiums. That is, the total income from premiums must significantly exceed the total payment for services.
4. Most office visits to medical professionals are fairly short. A Medscape survey (2018) found that the largest group of nonpsychiatric physicians reported visit lengths between 17 and 24 min.
5. There is an expectation that health providers, especially doctors, will provide biological treatment, e.g., medicines or surgery, and that they are not usually in the business of delivering training through structured curricula.
6. There is not usually a presumption that patients will do learning-based homework.
7. There is an assumption that positive results are dependent upon the quality of the treatment delivered, and not upon the extent and quality of work carried out by the patient.

All of these characteristics would lead us to predict that the distributions of time on task for psychotherapy more greatly resemble the distributions for medical visits than for schooling—which they do. Presumption 2 above would partially explain why psychotherapy would be often instituted only after maladaptive patterns had been practiced enough to develop significant habit strength, and only after some decrease in the quality of life had set in.

In summary, psychotherapy will probably not relieve the societal burden of psychopathology, because too small a fraction of people with psychopathology receive enough psychotherapy to make a difference.

References

Beck, J. S. (2021). *Cognitive behavior therapy: Basics and beyond* (3rd ed.). Guilford Press.

Bloom, B. S. (Ed.). (1985). *Developing talent in young people*. Ballantine Books.

Bruijniks, S. J. E., Lemmens, L. H. J. M., Hollon, S. D., Peeters, F. P. M. L., Cuijpers, P., Arntz, A., Dingemanse, P., Willems, L., van Oppen, P., Twisk, J. W. R., van den Boogaard, M., Spijker, J., Bosmans, J., & Huibers, M. J. H. (2020). The effects of once- versus twice-weekly sessions on psychotherapy outcomes in depressed patients. *The British Journal of Psychiatry., 216*(4), 222–230. https://doi.org/10.1192/bjp.2019.265

Bushnell, G. A., Dusetzina, S. B., Compton, S. N., Gaynes, B. N., Brookhart, M. A., & Stürmer, T. (2019). Psychotherapy claims surrounding pharmacotherapy initiation in children and adolescents with anxiety disorders. *Journal of Child and Adolescent Psychopharmacology, 29*(2), 100–106. https://doi.org/10.1089/cap.2018.0108

Chadwick, P. (2006). *Person-based cognitive therapy for distressing psychosis*. Wiley.

Code of Federal Regulations. (2026). Title 34. National Archives and Records Administration. https://www.ecfr.gov/current/title-34/subtitle-B/chapter-VI/part-600/subpart-A/section-600.2

Craig, T. K. J., Rus-Calafell, M., Ward, T., et al. (2018). AVATAR therapy for auditory verbal hallucinations in people with psychosis: A single-blind, randomised controlled trial. *The Lancet Psychiatry, 5*(1), 31–40.

Ericsson, A., & Pool, R. (2016). Malcolm Gladwell got us wrong: Our research was key to the 10,000-hour rule, but here's what got oversimplified. *Salon.* https://www.salon.com/2016/04/10/malcolm_gladwell_got_us_wrong_our_research_was_key_to_the_10000_hour_rule_but_heres_what_got_oversimplified/

Ericsson, K. A., Krampe, R. T., & Tesch-Römer, C. (1993). The role of deliberate practice in the acquisition of expert performance. *Psychological Review, 100*(3), 363–406. https://doi.org/10.1037/0033-295X.100.3.363

Flückiger, C., Wampold, B. E., Delgadillo, J., Rubel, J., Vîslă, A., & Lutz, W. (2020). Is there an evidence-based number of sessions in outpatient psychotherapy?—A comparison of naturalistic conditions across countries. *Psychotherapy and Psychosomatics, 89*(5), 333–335. https://doi.org/10.1159/000507793

Frank, E., Kupfer, D. J., Thase, M. E., et al. (2005). Two-year outcomes for interpersonal and social rhythm therapy in individuals with bipolar I disorder. *Archives of General Psychiatry, 62*(9), 996–1004.

Hincapie-Castillo, J. M., Liu, X., Bussing, R., & Winterstein, A. G. (2017). Prevalence of psychotherapy surrounding initiation of psychotropic polypharmacy in the Medicaid-insured population, 1999–2010. *Psychiatric Services, 68*(11), 1120–1126. https://doi.org/10.1176/appi.ps.201600511

Kazdin, A. E. (2005). *Parent management training: Treatment for oppositional, aggressive, and antisocial behavior in children and adolescents.* Oxford University Press.

Kazdin, A. E., & Blase, S. L. (2011). Rebooting psychotherapy research and practice to reduce the burden of mental illness. *Perspectives on Psychological Science, 6*, 21–37.

Kraft, M. A., & Novicoff, S. (2022). *Instructional time in U.S. public schools: Wide variation, causal effects, and lost hours* (EdWorkingPaper No. 22–652). Annenberg Institute at Brown University. https://files.eric.ed.gov/fulltext/ED625928.pdf

Lebowitz, E. R., Marin, C., Martino, A., Shimshoni, Y., & Silverman, W. K. (2020). Parent-based treatment as efficacious as cognitive-behavioral therapy for childhood anxiety: A randomized noninferiority study of supportive parenting for anxious childhood emotions. *Journal of the American Academy of Child and Adolescent Psychiatry, 59*(3), 362–372. https://doi.org/10.1016/j.jaac.2019.02.014

Lebowitz, E. R., & Shimshoni, Y. (2018). The SPACE program, a parent-based treatment for childhood and adolescent OCD: The case of Jasmine. *Bulletin of the Menninger Clinic, 82*(4), 266–287. https://doi.org/10.1521/bumc.2018.82.4.266

Lee, A. H., & DiGiuseppe, R. (2018). Anger and aggression treatments: A review of meta-analyses. *Current Opinion in Psychology, 19*, 65–74.

Linehan, M. M. (1993). *Cognitive-behavioral treatment of borderline personality disorder.* Guilford Press.

Medscape. (2018). *Medscape physician compensation report 2018.* https://www.medscape.com/slideshow/2018-compensation-overview-6009667

New York State Department of Motor Vehicles (2026). *Complete pre-licensing requirements.* https://dmv.ny.gov/driver-license/complete-pre-licensing-requirements

Saini, M. (2009). A meta-analysis of the psychological treatment of anger: Developing guidelines for evidence-based practice. *The Journal of the American Academy of Psychiatry and the Law, 37*(4), 473–488.

Schnurr, P. P., Friedman, M. J., Engel, C. C., Foa, E. B., Shea, M. T., Chow, B. K., Resick, P. A., Thurston, V., Orsillo, S. M., Haug, R., Turner, C., & Bernardy, N. (2007). Cognitive behavioral therapy for posttraumatic stress disorder in women: a randomized controlled trial. *JAMA, 297*(8), 820–830. https://doi.org/10.1001/jama.297.8.820

Shimshoni, Y., Silverman, W. K., & Lebowitz, E. R. (2020). SPACE-ARFID: A pilot trial of a novel parent-based treatment for avoidant/restrictive food intake disorder. *International Journal of Eating Disorders, 53*(10), 1623–1635. https://doi.org/10.1002/eat.23341

Strayhorn, J., Faraone, S. V., & Zhang-James, Y. (2025). Time on task limits psychotherapy's role in reducing the societal burden of aggression. *Frontiers in Public Health, 13*, 1570642. https://doi.org/10.3389/fpubh.2025.1570642

US Department of State, Foreign Service Institute. (2026). *Foreign language training*. https://www.state.gov/national-foreign-affairs-training-center/foreign-language-training

Wolpe, J. (1973). *The practice of behavior therapy* (2nd ed.). Pergamon Press.

Chapter 6
Psychoeducation, Contrasted with Psychotherapy

Abstract Depending on one's definitions, most psychotherapy is psychoeducation; that is, psychotherapy is a subset of psychoeducation. Psychotherapy aims to result in improved patterns of thought, feeling, and/or behavior as a result of experience, i.e., favorable learning. But psychoeducation can be carried out by other means that make it much more scalable. The more scalable forms of psychoeducation differ from psychotherapy in important ways. They are not dependent upon "medical necessity" and diagnosis of a disorder; thus, the stigma and the need for secrecy are reduced. Funding is not dependent upon insurance companies. The teachers don't need licensure within the health care system. The enterprise does not require the responsibility of measuring and mitigating dangerousness. Clients (or students) have more of an expectation that reading and doing written assignments are normative, and that informing someone about their lives (as in "talk therapy") is not the major method for improvement. There is much less time spent getting information from those being helped, and much more time delivering information to them. These forms of psychoeducation can sometimes be successfully carried out in groups or through mass-delivered means, more inexpensively than psychotherapy. If psychoeducation can be carried out in schools, time on task can be allocated without competing with everything else in life. If psychoeducation can be carried out early in life, preventively, there is a major advantage over waiting until skill deficiencies have created medical necessity for health care system involvement: the maladaptive patterns are not practiced for years before being addressed.

Keywords Psychoeducation · Psychological skills · Time on task · Nonprofessional · Scalability · Dangerousness · Preventive mental health · Medical insurance

Psychotherapy and psychoeducation share some important features. Both aim to improve mental health, to make positive changes in habitual patterns of thought, feeling, and behavior through experiences. In other words, both are influences that rely on learning. Both tend to make use of communication through language,

J. M. Strayhorn, Jr. et al., *The Promise of Psychoeducation in Relieving the Societal Burden of Psychopathology*, SpringerBriefs in Modern Perspectives on Disability Research, https://doi.org/10.1007/978-981-92-0922-4_1

although this is not a requirement: dogs and cats can benefit from desensitization procedures. Both aim toward improvement in psychological skills, although not all therapists would agree with the broad use of the word *skills* we employ. But both aim for improvement in such areas as forming positive relations with others, being productive, making good decisions on how to handle life situations, having emotional reactions to events that assist rather than hamper functioning, and so forth. Both rely on various methods of influence, which we will enumerate later. Both are greatly assisted by positive relationships between the learner and whoever is assisting the learning. Psychotherapy, as something meant to improve psychological skills by experience, can be regarded as a subset of psychoeducation.

But there are more scalable forms of psychoeducation that are different from psychotherapy in very important ways.

Psychotherapy is part of the health care system. In the USA at least, it is primarily paid for by medical insurance. In order for insurance to pay, there must be a claim of medical necessity, as justified by a diagnosis of a pathological condition. A great deal of importance is placed upon correct diagnosis, and diagnostic manuals (the International Classification of Diseases or the Diagnostic and Statistical Manual of the American Psychiatric Association) are referred to often; a diagnostic code is required for each session to be reimbursed by insurance. Much time and effort are put into discerning and documenting correct diagnoses. As with other health care professionals, psychotherapists must receive years of specialized education, pass licensing examinations, and obtain malpractice insurance. To practice without a license is a criminal offense. As with other health care providers, psychotherapists tend to practice during regular working hours; before the growth of telehealth, patients would need to transport themselves to offices during such hours.

Psychotherapy typically emphasizes the patient's talking about their life. Although research on how time is spent in psychotherapy sessions is very difficult to find, it's safe to say that a large fraction of the time is usually spent with the patient recounting what happened and with the therapist listening. Psychotherapy has been called "talk therapy." Many of the utterances therapists make are typically questions to the patient, directing the patient to talk more about a certain topic. Although some therapists make use of texts and manuals presenting a curriculum covered from start to finish, most of the time the patient comes to a therapy session with the agenda of talking about recent life experience, not of reviewing recent chapters of instruction, and certainly not taking tests over them. Psychotherapy usually does not include formal exercises meant to provide repetitive practice in psychological skills.

Psychotherapy is seldom delivered more than once a week. As we reviewed in the previous chapter, the number of visits and hours people typically complete in psychotherapy is dwarfed by the number of practices for an athletic team or the number of classes one has in math. If the entire population participated in many sessions of psychotherapy within the current system, funded by medical insurance, the costs of such would be impossibly high. Psychotherapists are often asked to produce results with people who are not willing to do any work between sessions, who are ambivalent or downright rejecting of change, or who are hostile to the entire enterprise; thus, a good bit of time can be spent in overcoming resistance and building relationships. Psychotherapy is much more often offered to adults and adolescents than to young children, i.e., those of the preschool and grade school years, despite the very important learnings that this age group is capable of when education is delivered well. Although the stigma of receiving mental health treatment has been reduced some in recent years, there remains an inevitable remnant of stigma in needing a mental health diagnosis to receive therapy. In keeping with this, privacy laws make for severe penalties for therapists who break confidentiality, for example by communicating that someone was in treatment, without that person's permission. Thus, on the one hand, practitioners should convey the attitude that there is nothing to be ashamed about in receiving psychotherapy; on the other hand, they must function in a climate where secrecy is the strictly enforced norm, and collaborate with patients with the assumption that such secrecy is desired. Whereas people put stickers on their cars and wear sweatshirts proudly proclaiming that they are an alumnus of X college, there is no market for stickers and sweatshirts proclaiming, "I'm a proud alumnus of psychotherapy with Dr. X." Accomplishments in learning math, gymnastics, music, dance, engineering, and so forth are advertised; accomplishments in learning emotional regulation, conflict-resolution, stress reduction, and so forth are kept secret. If a soccer coach sees a team member in a grocery store with others, social graces would dictate pleasant greetings and introductions. But if a psychotherapist sees a patient in a grocery store with others, passing by without giving any indication of recognition preserves the secrecy of their joint mission. Psychotherapists tend to view academic skills such as reading or math as in a totally separate bailiwick from other skills that make life better.

Psychoeducation can certainly be carried out within psychotherapy, and indeed, psychotherapy has been a major developing ground for how to impart psychological skills. But there are major differences as to how, when, and why psychoeducation may be delivered outside the psychotherapeutic relationship. Although psychotherapy is heterogeneous, psychoeducation is even more so: there are many settings and vehicles whereby it can be delivered. Anyone can buy a self-help book on psychological skills and educate themselves; anyone can find psychological self-help materials on the Internet. Parents can teach children the important principles of how to live well, without licenses or malpractice insurance. Peers can influence one another by educational methods, including modeling, reinforcement, and even instruction, sometimes without consciously setting out to do so. Nonprofessionals can teach children without automatically incurring liability for harmful behavior by the student. They can teach by reading with the learner, without having prior expertise in the content of the readings—they can learn along with the students. Skills can be taught and learned without the need for a diagnosis, but with a "transdiagnostic" philosophy: that all can benefit from learning about decision-making, handling stress, resolving conflict with others, the art of choosing one's own self-talk, adopting self-care habits, knowing the adverse effects of recreational drugs, and other skills. Classrooms of people, including children, can learn about psychological skills all at once. Older youth can be taught to read psychological skills instructions and practice exercises with younger children one-to-one. If teachers can make psychological skills exercises and writings fun for young children, the issue of "Are you motivated for this" can usually be bypassed—grade school children as a rule care more about whether the process of learning is interesting and fun than whether they have a prior wish to learn the content. School children are familiar with the set of norms wherein they are expected to do some work and where their performances in what they learn will be measured. They are familiar with the fact that learning takes time, and that many hours of work will be devoted to those subjects that are deemed most important. Psychoeducators in scalable programs, for example teachers of health or social and emotional learning in schools, do not take on the duty of doing detailed assessments for dangerousness. They do not need to spend time writing records for each child for each teaching session. They don't need to spend time on diagnosis. They are permitted and funded to teach psychological skills to those whose diagnosis is "normal." Unlike psychotherapists who, when they do explicitly teach, often ad lib their instructions, psychoeducators more typically use texts, manuals, and workbooks, relying on experts to create written communications read by students. There is no need for any sort of secrecy about the teaching enterprise, although rules still govern how an individual student's information is released. And there is no theoretical limitation to time on task.

Psychotherapists can be sued if their patients harm or kill themselves or others; therefore, an even higher priority for therapists than getting the patient better is making sure to cover the bases in evaluating and documenting dangerousness. In some clinics, therapists are expected to ask about suicidal and homicidal intent at every visit and to document the results. Psychotherapy is part of the health care system, and membership in that club brings with it what is indexed as "documentation burden." A survey of physicians revealed that more than a third spent 2 h or more outside of regular work hours on documentation; more than half felt that time spent documenting was inappropriately large (Gaffney et al., 2022). Tajirian et al. (2025) cited reports of twice as much time spent in documentation as in face-to-face contact. These researchers found, in physicians in a mental health organization, more than a quarter met criteria for burnout, and over half of those attributed burnout to the documentation burden. The imagined readership of such documentation includes billing and insurance auditors and potential malpractice attorneys. Such a system is not built for scalability in education.

Another major difference between psychoeducation and clinical mental health practice has to do with "upstream" versus "downstream" solutions. (These terms originated from the analogy of fixing a faulty bridge upstream versus rescuing people from the water downstream.) Many people enter the mental health treatment system only when things are so bad that suicidality is the presenting issue. Many people tolerate symptoms for many years before entering the clinical system; for example, it has been reported that the average adult patient presenting with obsessive-compulsive disorder had symptom onset at least 10 years before treatment onset (Rasmussen & Tsuang, 1986; Ziegler et al., 2021). Psychoeducation ideally should be delivered as a universal intervention, beginning as early in life as possible, with the goal of preventing "medical necessity" rather than waiting for it to develop and requiring it for services. This does not, however, mean that psychoeducation cannot be useful for those with the severest disorders.

The vision of high-quality schools where psychological skills form a major part of the curriculum, and where the culture and emotional climate of the school are carefully cultivated to maximize positive psychological development, is of course very attractive. But many schools are unfit places to teach psychological skills, for reasons including a very negative emotional climate. Such a climate can include hostile, defiant, bullying, and violent behaviors of students, the product of many environmental determinants; these maladaptive behaviors can coexist in a bidirectional causal loop with adversarial and harsh communications from teachers. Many schools are failing in the relatively straightforward task of teaching children to read; this does not raise hope for the more complex task of teaching people to be psychologically healthy. Many teachers have so many students to oversee at once that the main job is keeping control rather than educating. Teachers are often dealt classrooms with children of such disparate ability levels that it is difficult to avoid some of them feeling bored while others feel frustrated and confused. Many teachers are dealt a full classroom of children who are victims of adverse experiences in highly adverse neighborhoods, the education of most of whom might require very patient and prolonged one-to-one work. Schools sometimes devolve into institutions which exist primarily as a place where children can be kept while parents are at work. All this is certainly not meant to blame school personnel, who are mostly dedicated and kind people, who are often expected to do the impossible. But the point is that while excellent psychoeducation in schools is a very important goal for society, it is wise not to put all the eggs into the basket of formal schooling.

When we contrast psychotherapy with psychoeducation conducted elsewhere, the difference most relevant to societal burden is scalability. When nonprofessionals can pitch in to the task, when media such as books and videos can be fully employed, when groups of people can receive psychoeducation with no need for secrecy, and when psychoeducators do not need to take on the burden of continual review of diagnosis, assessment of dangerousness, and continual information-gathering and documentation regarding the client's or student's life, the possibilities for large-scale intervention are greatly enhanced.

References

Gaffney, A., Woolhandler, S., Cai, C., Bor, D., Himmelstein, J., McCormick, D., & Himmelstein, D. U. (2022). Medical documentation burden among US office-based physicians in 2019: A national study. *JAMA Internal Medicine, 182*(5), 564–566. https://doi.org/10.1001/jamainternmed.2022.0372

Rasmussen, S. A., & Tsuang, M. T. (1986). Clinical characteristics and family history in DSM-III obsessive-compulsive disorder. *American Journal of Psychiatry, 143*, 317–322.

Tajirian, T., Lo, B., Strudwick, G., Tasca, A., Kendell, E., Poynter, B., Kumar, S., Chang, P. B., et al. (2025). Assessing the impact on electronic health record burden after five years of physician engagement in a Canadian mental health organization: Mixed-methods study. *JMIR Human Factors, 12*, e65656. https://doi.org/10.2196/65656

Ziegler, S., Bednasch, K., Baldofski, S., & Rummel-Kluge, C. (2021). Long durations from symptom onset to diagnosis and from diagnosis to treatment in obsessive-compulsive disorder: A retrospective self-report study. *Plos One, 16*(12), e0261169. https://doi.org/10.1371/journal.pone.0261169

Chapter 7
A Psychological Skills Curriculum: What and How

Abstract In keeping with the definition of mental health, a psychoeducational curriculum works toward overarching goals of teaching people to be happy, to contribute to the happiness of others, and to be patient and resilient when the first two goals become elusive. This chapter presents a list of 62 psychological skills thought to contribute to the achievement of these goals; examples are awareness of one's own emotions, relaxation, option-generating, and tolerance of painful emotions. These can be organized into 16 groups, for example decision-making, fortitude, joyousness, and productivity. These may be taught or promoted by ten methods of influence, for example modeling, instruction, practice, and reinforcement. In addition to the skills of becoming mentally healthy oneself, the curriculum should include the study of how to make mental-health-friendly environments for both self and others. Such environments should include positive emotional climates, effort-payoff connection, quality models in media, and norms regarding substance use. A number of exercises are designed to give practice in psychological skills, involving for example celebrating one's positive examples of skills, fantasy rehearsing positive patterns, being a responsive listener, and brainstorming options for hypothetical situations. And excellent teaching in academic skills, particularly reading, is also of high priority.

Keywords Psychoeducational curriculum · Psychological skills · Mental-health-friendly environments · Social determinants · Parenting skills · Methods of influence · Modeling · Practice · Reinforcement · Instruction · Psychological skills exercises · Fantasy rehearsal · Reading skill

The enterprise of psychoeducation depends on answers to two questions: What do we want to teach? And how can we teach those things? If we could magically impart to people a set of skills or traits that would maximize their chances of psychological health, what should we choose to impart? Given that we can't do magic, what methods of influence really are available for this mission?

J. M. Strayhorn, Jr. et al., *The Promise of Psychoeducation in Relieving the Societal Burden of Psychopathology*, SpringerBriefs in Modern Perspectives on Disability Research, https://doi.org/10.1007/978-981-92-0922-4_1

7.1 Overarching Goals

A first agenda for psychoeducation is helping people orient themselves to overarching goals of happiness of self and happiness of others. Other ways of expressing this are kindness to self and kindness to others, caring for self and others, and loving our neighbors as ourselves. A third important goal is using fortitude and patience when the first two goals appear stymied. If we define mental health in this way, a first priority is to transmit this definition to students. There is some empirical information that goes along with these goals: the crucial idea that seeking one's own happiness and promoting the happiness of other people are goals that enhance each other, and are not in competition with one another. The correlation of "externalizing" and "internalizing" problems cited in Chap. 1 (correlations in the region of 0.3 to 0.5) is one type of empirical information about this.

Many adults and children consciously or unconsciously orient themselves toward far different goals. A major competitor is the goal of maximizing one's position on a dominance hierarchy, defeating one's adversaries. The child, or adult, who is intent on bullying, who gratuitously uses power to make others feel bad, and thereby demonstrates and sometimes shores up the power that comes from inducing fear, is an all too familiar example of the orientation toward power rather than happiness. Another major competitor is getting noticed, becoming famous. Among the tragic examples of this are people who have carried out acts of violence in order to become famous (Moore et al., 2023). A third competitor is the pursuit of short-term pleasure that detracts from more lasting happiness, as epitomized by seeking euphoric effects of drugs and alcohol, but also exemplified by unwise practices of eating, electronic entertainment, thrill-seeking, or sexual activity. And a fourth is the seeking of material wealth, of increasing one's net financial worth, without regard to the effects on human happiness. Exemplars might be those who become rich from marketing of cigarettes, gambling, violent entertainment, or social media that prove harmful to society.

7.2 Psychological Skills

What are the skills that enable people to be happy and to make others happy?

One of us (JMS) has spent much time over several decades, asking the question, in case after case of clinical psychiatric practice, and in reported cases and reported psychotherapeutic methods, "What could (or did) this person learn to do better, to enhance the quality of life?" (Strayhorn, 1983, 1988). The same question has been asked of writings in the fields of religion and philosophy that suggest competences that make life better. The goal has been to compile a fairly comprehensive list of the skills contributing to mental health.

Why compile such a list? First, with respect to psychotherapy, it provides a "diagnostic axis" that is more relevant to learning-based remediation than is traditional symptom and syndrome-based diagnosis. For example, suppose two people are depressed. One gives lots of evidence of being depressed because of loneliness, and great difficulty in meeting people and building relationships with them. A second is capable of friendship-building, but gives lots of evidence of being extremely self-critical and lacking in self-reinforcing cognitions. If one is making decisions about drug treatment, they both might get the same drug by virtue of similar symptoms. But if one is devising learning-based treatment, teaching social skills and desensitizing social fears with the first, and teaching self-reinforcement and self-forgiveness to the second would be quite different strategies that the "skills axis diagnoses" would suggest.

A second reason for compiling such a list is that it can form a curriculum outline for preventive mental health. If we know which skills produce mental health, ideally we construct readings, activities, practice exercises, and measures for each one of them, and place high priority on each individual receiving adequate training in each of them.

The "skills axes" referred to earlier have been through several revisions; the following is the most current.

Psychological Skills Axis

Group 1: Productivity

1. Purposefulness. Having a sense of purpose that drives activity.
2. Persistence. Sustaining attention, concentrating, focusing, staying on task.
3. Competence-development. Working toward competence in job, academics, recreation, life skills.
4. Organization. Organizing goals, priorities, time, money, and physical objects; planfulness.

Group 2. Joyousness

5. Enjoying aloneness. Having a good time by oneself, tolerating not getting someone's attention.
6. Pleasure from approval. Enjoying approval, compliments, and positive attention from others.
7. Pleasure from accomplishments. Self-reinforcement for successes.
8. Pleasure from your own kindness. Feeling pleasure from doing kind, loving acts for others.
9. Pleasure from discovery. Enjoying exploration and satisfaction of curiosity.
10. Pleasure from others' kindness. Feeling gratitude for what others have done.
11. Pleasure from blessings. Celebrating and feeling the blessings of luck or fate.
12. Pleasure from affection. Enjoying physical affection without various fears interfering.
13. Favorable attractions. Having feelings of attraction aroused in ways consonant with happiness.
14. Gleefulness. Playing, becoming childlike, experiencing glee, being spontaneous.
15. Humor. Enjoying funny things, finding and producing comedy in life.

Group 3: Kindness

16. Kindness. Nurturing someone, being kind and helpful.
17. Empathy. Recognizing other people's feelings, seeing things from the other's point of view.
18. Conscience. Feeling appropriate guilt, avoiding harming others.

Group 4: Honesty

19. Honesty. Being honest and dependable, especially when it's difficult to be so.
20. Awareness of your own abilities. Being honest and brave in assessing your strengths and weaknesses.

Group 5: Fortitude

21. Frustration-tolerance. Handling frustration, tolerating adverse circumstances, fortitude.
22. Handling separation. Tolerating separation from close others, or loss of a relationship.
23. Handling rejection. Tolerating it when people don't like or accept you, or don't want to be with you.
24. Handling criticism. Dealing with disapproval, criticism and lack of respect from others.
25. Handling mistakes and failures. Regretting mistakes without being overly self-punitive.
26. Magnanimity, non-jealousy. Handling it when someone else gets what you want.
27. Painful emotion-tolerance. Avoiding "feeling bad about feeling bad".
28. Fantasy-tolerance. Tolerating mental images of unwanted behavior, confident that you will not enact them.

Group 6: Good decisions
6a: Individual decision-making

29. Positive aim. Aiming toward making things better. Seeking reward and not punishment.
30. Thinking before acting. Thinking, rather than responding impulsively or by reflex, when it's useful to do so.
31. Verbal fluency. Using words to conceptualize the world: verbal skills.
32. Awareness of your emotions. Recognizing, and being able to verbalize your own feelings.
33. Awareness of control. Accurately assessing the degree of control you have over specific events.
34. Decision-making. Defining a problem, gathering information, generating options, predicting and evaluating consequences, making a choice.

6b: Joint decision-making, including conflict resolution

35. Toleration. Non-bossiness. Tolerating a wide range of other people's behavior.
36. Rational approach to joint decisions. Deciding rationally on stance and strategies for joint decisions.
37. Option-generating. Generating creative options for solutions to problems.

38. Option-evaluating. Justice skills: Recognizing just solutions to interpersonal problems.
39. Assertion. Dominance, sticking up for yourself, taking charge, enjoying winning.
40. Submission: Conciliation, giving in, conceding, admitting one was wrong, being led.
41. Differential reinforcement. Reinforcing positive behavior and avoiding reinforcing the negative.

Group 7: Nonviolence

42. Forgiveness and anger control. Forgiving. Handling and enacting rational responses to an insult or injury by another.
43. Nonviolence. Being committed to the principle of nonviolence and working to foster it.
1. Group 8: Respectful talk, not being rude.
44. Respectful talk, not being rude. Being sensitive to words, vocal tones, and facial expressions that are accusing, punishing, or demeaning, and avoiding them unless there is a very good reason.

Group 9: Friendship-Building

45. Discernment and Trusting. Accurately appraising others. Not distorting with prejudice, overgeneralization, wish-fulfilling fantasies, projections, or transference from previous interpersonal encounters. Deciding what someone can be trusted for, and trusting when appropriate.
46. Self-disclosure. Disclosing and revealing oneself to another when it's safe.
47. Gratitude. Expressing gratitude, admiration, and other positive feelings toward others.
48. Social interaction. Starting social interaction; engaging well in social conversation or play; listening well; using tones of enthusiasm and approval; knowing what is "appropriate," and not, to say and do.
49. Reasonable expectations. Not having unreasonably high expectations from relationships; not feeling too entitled. At the same time, being able to insist on being treated justly; not tolerating abusive or unreasonable behavior from the other.
50. Sending and receiving value messages. Being able to communicate to the other that they, and the relationship, are valued, through channels that the other can receive; being able to receive another's value messages.

Group 10: Self-discipline

51. Self-discipline. Delay of gratification, self-control. Denying yourself present pleasure for future gain.

Group 11: Loyalty

52. Loyalty. Tolerating and enjoying sustained closeness, attachment, and commitment to another, keeping commitments to others. Repairing rifts in relationships. But also deciding when not to give unfair advantage to your friends or relatives, and deciding whom you don't owe loyalty to.

Group 12: Conservation

53. Conservation and Thrift. Preserving resources for ourselves and future generations. Not wasting time, money, or the earth's resources.

Group 13: Self-care

54. Carefulness. Feeling appropriate fear and avoiding unwise risks.
55. Habits of self-care. Healthy habits regarding drinking, smoking, drug use, exercise, diet, noise exposure, sleep, sun exposure, auto safety, fire safety, exposure to infections, and others.
56. Relaxation. Calming yourself, relaxing muscles, meditating, lowering the level of arousal when warranted.
57. Self-nurture. Delivering assuring or care-taking thoughts to yourself, feeling comforted thereby; choosing behaviors that care for yourself.

Group 14: Compliance

58. Compliance. Obeying, submitting to legitimate and reasonable authority. Doing your part for the rule of law. But also deciding when to disobey misguided commands or rules.

Group 15: Positive fantasy rehearsal

59. Imagination and positive fantasy rehearsal. Using fantasy as a tool in rehearsing or evaluating a plan, or adjusting to an event or situation. Avoiding entertaining yourself with violent images.

Group 16: Courage

60. Courage. Estimating danger, overcoming fear of non-dangerous situations, handling danger rationally.
61. Depending. Accepting help, being dependent without shame, asking for help appropriately.
62. Independent thinking. Making decisions independently, carrying out actions independently.

For most direct work with students or patients, the names of the groups give sufficient detail, without being so burdensome upon memory. The following is the short version of the psychological skills list:

1. Productivity. Work toward worthy goals.
2. Joyousness. Mentally celebrate your good luck, the beneficial things others have done, and your own good choices.
3. Kindness. Try to make other people happier.
4. Honesty. Tell the truth; avoid cheating and stealing.
5. Fortitude. Handle it when you don't get what you want.
6. Good individual decisions. Think carefully about what to do, especially in important choice points.

7. Good joint decisions, including conflict resolution. Talk calmly and think rationally when making joint decisions and when your wishes seem to conflict with someone else's.
8. Nonviolence. Don't hurt or kill. Work toward a nonviolent world.
9. Respectful talk. Choose your words so as to promote good feelings, rather than to punish or humiliate, unless there is a very good reason for exception.
10. Friendship-building. Build good relations with people.
11. Self-discipline. Choose actions that accomplish worthy goals and produce long-term happiness, even when they don't bring the most pleasure at the moment.
12. Loyalty. Make good choices about keeping commitments to people and sticking up for those who have been good to you.
13. Conservation. Conserve, rather than waste, time, money, and the earth's resources.
14. Self-care. Look after your health and safety, as well as that of others.
15. Compliance. Support the rule of law; obey reasonable and just authority. Make careful decisions about when it is right to disobey.
16. Positive fantasy rehearsal. Use imagination to practice doing admirable things. Avoid entertaining yourself with violent images.
17. Courage. Be brave enough to do what's best.

Each of the skills can be the subject of instruction through positive models and expository writing; each of them can be practiced by psychological skills exercises. It has been a decades-long project of one of us (JMS) to produce such teaching materials. Many exercises tend to strengthen more than one skill: for example, the reflections exercise, where the learner practices responding to utterances of the preceptor with empathic paraphrases, is meant to develop both concentration skills and social conversation skills. The twelve-thought exercise, where the learner practices making up 12 different categories of thoughts about the same situation, contributes to joyousness, fortitude, decision-making, and several others that are helped by good choices of self-talk.

The categorization of skills listed above is certainly not the only one that has been constructed or that could be constructed. There is much in common with virtues or ethical principles or positive psychological patterns as listed or included in writings by Aristotle, Benjamin Franklin, Cognitive Behavior Therapy, Dialectical Behavior Therapy, Positive Psychology theorists, The Scout Law, the Jewish or Christian Bibles, the Tao Te Ching, the Analects of Confucius, the Unitarian Universalist Principles, skills of Aggression Replacement Training, the principles of the Heartwood Ethics Program, social skills training programs, and probably many others.

7.3 Constructing Mental-Health-Friendly Environments

Earlier, we made the points that environmental factors are major contributors to mental health, that the most important environmental influences are supplied by other people, and that therefore one person's learned habits become part of another person's environment. Thus, a major part of psychoeducation should include that subset of kindness that has to do with how to construct mental-health-friendly environments for other people. This implies that part of the agenda of psychoeducation is the study of the question, what constitutes a mental-health-friendly environment? And how can each of us contribute to the mental-health-friendliness of any environments we can influence? Below are some of the environmental factors that are components of a mental-health-friendly environment.

1. A favorable physical environment, including non-toxicity and protection from infection.

Even decades after the discovery that lead is neurotoxic, in much lower amounts than previously realized, there are still children whose learning is being impaired by environmental lead. Cadmium, nanoplastics, mercury, pesticides—freeing our brains and our bodies from these is a high priority for humanity. Likewise, eliminating the harm done by toxocara (roundworms) infections, tuberculosis, HIV, and other preventable infections is high on the agenda—mental health exists in a context of physical health. Opportunities for silence and solitude are other favorable aspects of the physical environment. A physical environment conducive to adequate sleep, including one free of too much noise, is important.

2. Opportunity for human connection, versus loneliness (Kraav et al., 2021; Park et al., 2020; Wilkialis et al., 2021).

Institutions and cultural practices that help people to get to know one another, to form positive relationships, foster mental health.

3. Friendly, kind, nonviolent behavior.

The absence of cruelty, and kindness, in families are conducive to mental health (Ogbaselase et al., 2022; Burkhouse et al., 2012). Kind, not verbally abusive, nonviolent behavior in schools (Wolke et al., 2013; Copeland et al., 2013), workplaces (Gray et al., 2019), neighborhoods (Jackson et al., 2019), and between nations (Carpiniello, 2023) is important. War and the impending threat of war are sources of trauma and anxiety that are hard to overestimate. Cruelty based on prejudice and discrimination against groups other than one's own has been a scourge of humanity and a major contributor to mental disorder.

4. Positive emotional climates.

These are outgrowths of kindness among people in the social system. In a positive emotional climate, the ratio of approving to disapproving utterances is high; there is a feeling of trust and security that people have the others' best interests at heart as well as their own; there is a prevailing feeling of cooperation rather than adversarial interaction; people tend to enjoy doing things with each other; matters can be discussed openly; there is no need for deception and secrecy.

5. An effort-payoff connection.

This refers to being able to attain positive payoffs, or reinforcers, contingent upon efforts. This is the opposite of learned helplessness, where there is not a contingent relationship between efforts and rewards (Carvalho & Hopko, 2011; Abramson et al., 1978).

6. Employment.

The availability of decent and meaningful jobs is an important aspect of the effort-payoff connection (McGee & Thompson, 2015). Gerald Patterson and colleagues produced major improvements in children's behavior by programs which included (among several other components) helping parents arrange contingent reinforcement for children's performing chores—otherwise describable as giving them a job (Patterson, 1975).

7. The match of challenge level and skill level.

A match between skill levels and challenge levels appears crucial to well-being, (Csikszentmihalyi, 1990). The more schools and jobs can provide challenges commensurate with current abilities, the greater well-being is predicted. Part of the art of providing this environmental factor involves having training programs in place where people can start at a comfortable place on the hierarchy of difficulty and move upward.

8. Opportunities for meaning and purpose.

Frankl (2006) emphasized the search for meaning and purpose as crucial components of good life. In keeping with this, it's desirable that the jobs the culture offers, and the subjects of study and the activities the schools offer, provide a sense of doing something really worthwhile—that is, something that increases the net happiness of the world.

9. Norms regarding addictive drugs.

As would be expected, addiction and depression are comorbid (Xu et al., 2020; NIDA, 2018); the use of addictive substances is comorbid with almost all types of psychopathology. Cultural norms that encourage sobriety enhance mental health.

10. Availability of psychoeducation.

If the learnings accumulated through psychotherapy are available and delivered routinely, mental health should be advanced (Eiraldi et al., 2016a, 2016b), as we will discuss in more detail.

11. The models present in media.

Many children spend much more time in consuming mass media than they spend doing schoolwork or being with parents (Rideout et al., 2010; Rideout & Robb, 2019; Rideout et al., 2022). The effect of mass media on mental health has been studied vigorously (e.g., Haidt, 2024; Anderson et al., 2017). But the availability and the content of electronic entertainment is determined more by the marketplace than by scientific study of what is helpful. How much political and racial hatred is stirred up through the mass media, versus how much the media mobilize a wish to help one's fellow citizens, is difficult to estimate.

12. Poverty, and its relief.

Depression is related to socioeconomic status (Galea et al., 2005; Ridley et al., 2020). How can a society provide ways, especially for those at the lower end of the socioeconomic scale, to get basic needs met, do meaningful work, earn livable wages, and have time for positive relationships? The correlates of poverty may be more harmful than low income itself: living in a neighborhood with high crime, violence, drug use, unemployment, and failing schools.

13. Stewardship of the earth's environment.

Global climate change is of course one of the major challenges facing humanity. The threats to mental health springing from it include not just hotter temperatures, but major social disruptions (Peñuelas & Nogué, 2023). Pollution, destruction of animal habitats, and other threats to the liveability of the planet are serious challenges. In the ideal mental-health-friendly environment, wishes to contribute to the solutions to these problems are stimulated and harnessed.

14. Access to nature.

Evidence indicates that part of a mental-health-friendly environment is having access to being in nature (Jimenez et al., 2021; Bettmann et al., 2024).

15. Good government.

Various aspects of governmental policy are associated with more positive mental health outcomes (McCartney et al., 2019). Government that is non-corrupt, that promotes the rule of reasonable law, and whose leaders model kindness, nonviolence, respectful talk, honesty, and other psychological skills is a contributor to mental health. Government that is responsive to the needs and wishes of the governed, and that operates with the consent of and in the best interests of the governed, is important. The rule of law provided by government provides nonviolent methods of dispute resolution when the individuals involved fail at this. These aspects of governance are important whether the person doing the governing is a president, a chief executive officer, a boss in charge of two employees, a teacher in charge of a classroom, or a parent governing or co-governing a household.

16. Availability of weapons.

Nations, localities, and families vary widely in the degree of ownership of firearms, and the rates of violence are correlated (Siegel et al., 2013). Exposure to the use of weapons of destruction in warfare, even without actual injury, is unsurprisingly associated with long-lasting adverse mental health effects (Morganstein et al., 2023).

17. Expectations for positive achievement.

In the mental-health-friendly environment, the culture values and reinforces achievements that contribute to the well-being of society (and not just those that succeed in grabbing the most of its attention). Expectations will need to be adjusted according to the talents of the individuals, but there is also an expectation that society will find ways to elicit positive achievements and useful contributions from almost all people, for the good of the contributor as well as that of society.

18. Training, so as to reduce the need for punishment.

Much of the world runs on influencing people by making rules and then punishing those who do not follow the rules. The more people can be taught why certain behavior patterns are desirable and how to do them skillfully, the less punishment is needed. As one example, there are various thoughtfully created manuals on nonviolent conflict-resolution and anger control (e.g., Glick & Gibbs, 2011; Rosenberg, 2015; Strayhorn, 2006). Of the people being punished for violence, it is safe to bet that almost none of them have been thoroughly exposed to the content of such manuals, and even fewer have thoroughly practiced the skills and exercises therein. As another example, children are punished for not doing well in school, without having been taught systematically how to study, and sometimes without being taught well how to read.

These defining aspects of a mental-health-friendly environment are applicable on both the macro and the micro level. From a relationship between two people to humanity as a whole, including workplaces, classrooms, community organizations, and families, mental health will be enhanced by these aspects. This list could be considerably enlarged. But if these eighteen aspects of the environment were magically made extremely favorable, the effect on society would be enormous—possibly greater than all that the health care system does for mental health. Contemporary society is not doing well in these regards, and past societies probably did even worse.

Part of the thesis of this book is that psychoeducation that includes much study and thought about environmental determinants of mental health may greatly improve progress. How do the most important characteristics of the environment get created? People learn habits that enhance or detract from other people's environments. The improvement of the mental health environment must come from people's learning to provide good environments for others. All aspects of creating positive environments can be, and should be, the subjects of psychoeducation.

7.4 Parents, Family Members, and Relationship Members, as Designers of Mental-Health-Friendly Environments

Many of the aspects of the mental-health-friendly culture require collective action of many people. But each family, and each relationship between or among any number of people, including a dyad, is its own micro-environment. Each person has the chance to contribute to a more mental-health-friendly environment in their own relationships.

Parent training is a thoroughly tested and highly efficacious intervention (Leijten et al., 2016, 2019). There is one catch for parent training, however: of all the people in society, parents tend to have the least amount of discretionary time to devote to parent training. When free parenting classes have been widely publicized, only a small fraction of parents have elected to participate. But the behaviors that constitute good parenting overlap greatly with those of having good relationships of other sorts, including good relationships between a tutor and a student, or between friends. Below are some of the aspects of positive micro-environments that may be part of a psychoeducational curriculum. These overlap considerably with the more general list given above, but they are important enough to justify a little repetition. These are written from the point of view of one person, to emphasize that individuals often (but not always) have unilateral power to improve the emotional climate of relationships:

1. Opportunity for connection.

   Does the person in the relationship spend time with and pay attention to the other?

2. Models of kindness.

   Does the person show kind and caring behaviors toward the other?

3. Reinforcement of the other person's positive examples.

   Does the person notice the other person's positive examples of psychological skills, and celebrate them, by compliments, thank-yous, attention, enthusiastic tones of voice, and remembering the positive example and mentioning it later? This has been identified as one of the common elements of successful parent training.

4. Non-reinforcement of negative behavior.

   When the other person is doing something unpleasant, the person thinks twice about the strategy of doing what they want to get them to stop. (Sometimes, when what the person wants is completely reasonable, it's rational to reward protest that isn't experienced as pleasant.)

5. Non-bossiness.

   Particularly in parenting relationships, there is a need for some commands given. But unnecessary commands should be eliminated. It's important to clearly differentiate commands and suggestions. Parents should follow up with commands that they do give, and reinforce compliance.

6. REFFF versus CCCT.

   The letters stand for different type of verbalizations. R = reflections. "What I hear you saying is ____." E = Telling about your own experience. "Want to hear about a choice I had to make today?..." F=Facilitations. "Uh huh. Yes. I see. Oh? OK. Humh..." F = Follow up questions. "What happened next? Tell me more, please." F = Positive Feedback. "Thanks for doing that." "I'm glad you told me about that." "Sounds like a good idea."

With CCCT on the other hand: C=Commands. "Stop doing that. Come here, now." Criticisms: "That was a selfish and bratty thing for you to do." Contradictions: "No, you've got it wrong. That's not the way it is at all." T = Threats. "If you keep doing that, I'm going to retaliate in this way…"

Some use of CCCT is necessary in parenting, and in most other relationships. So it's not a matter of completely eliminating these utterances, but of keeping the relative frequency low. It has been recommended that the ratio of approving to disapproving utterances be 4 to 1 or greater for positive relationships.

The use of less aversive, more reinforcing and rational verbalizations, makes for a more positive emotional climate.

7. Positive models.

The models of behavior coming into the system are ideally skewed as much as possible toward positive examples of psychological skills. For parenting, this implies accomplishing the difficult feat of helping children avoid violent entertainment.

8. Mutually gratifying activities.

The people in the relationship look for ways of doing things together that are gratifying, fun, fulfilling, for both. Can they enjoy walking and talking together? Enjoy doing chores together? Taking turns reading aloud to each other? Playing cooperative games? Singing or dancing together? Doing sports activities?

9. Dr. L.W. Aap.

The letters Dr. L.W. Aap are a mnemonic for steps in joint decision-making or conflict resolution. D = Defining the choice point. They each define the situation they are in and their own interests, without blaming the other. R = Reflecting. They each paraphrase the problem definition they heard from the other, to make sure they understand it correctly. L = Listing. They list options for courses of action. W=Waiting. They wait until they are finished listing before they start evaluating the options. A = Advantages. They evaluate the options by speaking about the positive and negative consequences of them, i.e., the advantages and disadvantages (and not by speaking about the bad aspects of the other person's personality). A = Agreeing. They agree on some plan, even if it's only to think some more and reconvene later. P=Politeness. They speak with courtesy throughout.

It is usually impossible to come close to Dr. L.W. Aap when one or both people is at least moderately angry. An important part of the conflict resolution process is that either person should be able to postpone communication and for the two people to go to separate rooms and stop interacting and cool off, without the other person getting further inflamed by this. If this rule by itself were followed, a great deal of domestic violence could probably be prevented.

7.5 How to Teach? The Methods of Influence Axis

In order to influence behavior, legislatures make laws; if people break the laws, they are punished. Schools have rules against various types of misbehavior, and apply punishments when rules are broken. Parents "discipline" or punish children for misbehavior. Nations are ready to influence the behavior of other nations by readiness to punish them via armies and weapons. It appears that punishment is one of the major ways that people rely on to try to elicit positive behaviors from others. But there are other means by which people can influence one another, and the psychological skills curriculum should both use these methods in its own teaching, and teach these methods to students to use in their lives. Here are ten methods of influence, of which punishment is only a small part. These are discussed more in Strayhorn (1988):

1. Objective-formation.

   Helping someone decide that a certain behavior pattern is desirable for them. The use of motivational interviewing is an example of interaction that promotes objective-formation.

2. Hierarchy.

   The word hierarchy is shorthand for devising a hierarchy of tasks or challenges that one can move along, on the way toward increased competence. Just as one starts on the road to piano expertise by playing Twinkle, Twinkle, Little Star instead of Rachmaninoff's 3rd Concerto, one starts on the road to courage skills by something other than thrusting oneself immediately into the real-life feared situation.

3. Relationship.

   Having a positive relationship with a person increases the strength of influence the person can have.

4. Attribution.

   The influencing person attributes to the other the power to change rather than looking at the other's traits as fixed.

5. Modeling.

   People tend to imitate the behavior they see and hear, whether the models are positive or negative.

6. Practice.

   Repetitive practice of positive patterns can produce amazing changes in the brain, as evidenced by those who have used repetitive practice to become virtuosos in music, sports, or other fields; repetitive practice could be much more widely harnessed in the service of psychological skill development. Fantasy rehearsal is an important subset of practice methods.

7. Reinforcement and punishment contingencies.

We tend to repeat those behaviors that result in desirable consequences and avoid those that result in lack of desired consequences or undesirable consequences. Self-reinforcing thoughts are an important subset of reinforcers.

8. Instruction.

Someone uses words or pictures or videos to teach you how to do the behavior in question.

9. Stimulus control.

For example: it's easier to avoid alcohol if you stay out of bars; it's easier to avoid wasting time doom-scrolling if you are working at a place without an Internet connection; it's easier to start practicing your musical instrument if it's nearby and handy; it's easier to do academic work if you're one-to-one with a tutor than if you're in a classroom with highly distracting peers.

10. Monitoring.

Just as it's easier to gain competence as a basketball shooter if you can see whether your shots go in, it's easier to gain competence almost all other skills if you can get feedback on your progress. The use of biofeedback to monitor progress in relaxation and lowering the flight-or-fight response is one of many possible examples.

7.6 The Concept of Psychological Skills Exercises

We would be very unlikely to devise a math course without providing practice problems for students to solve; we'd be very unlikely to coach a basketball team without providing practice of the maneuvers of shooting, passing, guarding, dribbling, and so forth. Whenever one is learning a skill, it is helpful, if not essential, to practice that skill repeatedly. And so it is with psychological skills. But how can psychological skills be practiced? Real life, of course, offers opportunities to practice those skills. But the practice opportunities of real life often come when we are overloaded with other demands, when a response is demanded too quickly, or when we are caught off guard. It is possible to engineer methods for deliberate practice of psychological skills at times when performance is likely to be of desirable patterns. Such methods may be called psychological skills exercises, and the following are some of them. They will be described as if carried out in tutoring, although they can be carried out in other types of groups. These are a subset of a much larger number described by Strayhorn (2001, 2013).

The Celebrations Exercise

The two people take turns answering two questions: (1) what's something you're glad that you did and (2) which psychological skills was that an example of? For example, the tutor says, "Let's do the celebrations exercise! I'll go first. This morning instead of sitting down and doing some doomscrolling right after getting up, I did a little exercise and then did some things on my to do list. I think that was self-care, self-discipline, and productivity. Your turn!"

The purpose of this exercise is to harness the power of self-reinforcement for one's positive actions, and to harness the power of fantasy rehearsal that is implicit in the act of calling those actions to consciousness another time.

Skills Stories

This exercise is like the celebrations exercise, only instead of remembering a positive example, the person makes up a positive example, and identifies the skills exemplified. A variant is taking turns making up skills stories for each of the skills, in order.

The Brainstorming Options Exercise

The two people take turns thinking of possible options for a choice point. Example: "The choice point is that someone in a school sees another student being verbally bullied by another student. Let's take turns thinking of options; I'll go first. The person could talk with the student who is being bullied, and find out more about what their experience is. Your turn!"

A great deal of research has found that the ability to generate options is positively correlated with mental health, that the skill of generating options is teachable, and that teaching this skill leads to improvements in mental health (Chang et al., 2004).

The Divergent Thinking Exercise

The two people take turns generating answers to a question that can be answered in many ways. For example, the question is: A person feels proud of themselves. What did they do to make them feel proud? Or: A person forgot something. What did they forget?

The brainstorming options exercise is a subset of the divergent thinking exercise; the divergent thinking exercise is a great preparatory step.

The Pros and Cons Exercise

The two people take turns generating advantages or disadvantages in the form of positive or negative consequences of a certain option. For example, the option is, "A person considers adopting a pet dog."

Listing pros and cons has been a part of cognitive behavior therapy and motivational interviewing. It is basic to decision-making. It was famously recommended by one of the fathers of psychological self-help, Benjamin Franklin (1772).

The Reflections Exercise

One person speaks, and stops talking often. Each time the first stops, the second responds with a reflection: "What I hear you saying is ___," or "If I understand you right, ____" or the like. This exercises both concentration skills and skills of listening useful in social conversation.

Listening with Four Responses

One person speaks, and each time they stop, the second practices a response chosen from one of the following four types of utterances: a reflection, a facilitation (such as, I see, OK, yes…), a follow-up question, or positive feedback. In real-life social conversation, if someone does reflections with every utterance, the other is likely to think them very unusual; if they vary between the four responses done well, the other is likely to think that they are a good listener.

The Tones of Approval Exercise

The student practices discriminating and classifying when the tutor models utterances in tones of voice that are neutral, of small to moderate approval and enthusiasm, or of large approval and enthusiasm. Then the tutor provides an utterance and a degree of approval for the student to enact. Example: "Can you say, 'You got that right' with small to moderate approval?"

In social interaction, tones of voice are a very important way of making the other person feel valued.

The Twelve-Thought Exercise

The tutor and student pick a situation, and then take turns generating each of 12 types of thoughts about that same situation. Example: The situation is that I had an appointment to meet someone, but they don't show up and their phone goes to voice mail. Twelve thoughts: (1) Awfulizing—Oh no, maybe something horrible has happened to them! (2) Getting down on myself—I just don't seem to elicit respect from people. (3) Blaming someone else—They are so inconsiderate to stand me up! (4) Not awfulizing—They probably just forgot; this isn't the end of the world. (5) Not getting down on myself—I've been gentle with people when they do things like this, and maybe that makes them less scared of standing me up, but I don't want to punish myself for being kind and forgiving. (6) Not blaming someone else—They probably just forgot; I've forgotten things myself; I don't want to come down on them too hard. (7) Goal-setting—My goals are to have a reasonable response to the other person, and to figure out something else to do during this time. (8) Listing options and choosing—I could suggest to the other person that they use an appointment calendar to organize. I could leave a voice mail saying looks like you can't make the appointment; I'll see you another time. I could just wait a little longer and leave and let them get in touch with me. I could leave a voice mail asking if they had the same time planned for this as I did. In the time that is freed up, I could do some work on my to do list, go for a walk, or just goof off and relax. I think I'll ask by voice mail if they had this time down like I did and then go for a walk. (9) Learning from the experience—Maybe in the future I'll text people to remind them of appointments, if I think of it. (10) Celebrating luck—I'm lucky that nothing worse than this has happened to me today, or lately. (11) Celebrating someone else's choice—I feel good about all the people who have showed up on time for appointments with me. (12) Celebrating my own choice—I am glad I stayed cool about this and didn't act out anger toward the other person and thought of something good to do instead.

This exercise is an educational condensation of cognitive therapy; it is meant to help people choose their own self-talk. There is no one of the 12 thoughts that should be avoided altogether; people cause themselves trouble by overdoing or overgeneralizing the first three. Sometimes it's useful to think of examples which do, and do not, overdo those.

By doing this exercise, people strengthen their cognitive flexibility—their ability to pick the type of self-talk that is most useful for them in any given situation, rather than being stuck in habits. This helps with skills of joyousness, fortitude, good decisions, and most other psychological skills.

The Four-Thought Exercise

It takes a while to generate each of the 12 thoughts in real life. The four-thought exercise allows practice of a subset of the 12 thoughts, to give practice in a default way of responding to unwanted situations, for example those that might trigger anger or fear. The four thoughts are not awfulizing, goal setting, listing options and choosing, and celebrating your own choice. Example: I'm driving the speed limit, and someone honks at me and gestures aggressively at me for not going fast enough. Not awfulizing: Nothing harmful has happened. Goal-setting: My goal is to stay cool and not have things escalate. I'd like for there to be only one person who is very upset rather than two. Listing and choosing: I could find a place to pull over at the side of the road or into a business parking lot and let this person pass. I could relax my muscles to help myself not be upset. I think I'll do both of those. Celebrating my own choice: Hooray, I made a good choice, and I did a good practice of nonviolence and anger control.

STEBC Fantasy Rehearsals

In this, someone describes a Situation, and decides upon and describes the Thoughts, Emotions, and Behaviors that they think are the best way of handling the situation, and then practices Celebrating handling the situation well. For example, someone has something of a symmetry compulsion, and wastes time getting socks exactly the same height. Situation: I deliberately arrange my socks so that one is lower than the other. Thoughts: If I can get used to this, I'll really have reason to feel good. Emotions: I feel a SUD (subjective units of distress) level, but I also feel determined to have a success and I feel proud of myself for taking this on. Behaviors: I leave my socks like this and go on with my day. Every once in a while I remember this, and I notice that my SUD level is going way down. Celebration: Hooray, this is a courage skills triumph for me, and it represents lots of progress in something important!

This is an example of a "coping" rehearsal, where the situation causes some negative emotion, but the person does what's best anyway. In a "mastery" rehearsal, one imagines that either by a miracle or by diligent work, the situation has become no problem at all, and one can handle it without any SUD level.

Fantasy rehearsals can help with practice of any psychological skill. One variation is to write out fantasy rehearsals and to read them daily.

Joint Decision Role-Play, or Dr. L.W. Aap

Two people each play a part, or one person plays both parts, for two people who are making a joint decision in a choice point. They each (1) *Define* the problem without blaming or commanding the other. (2) *Reflect* to make sure they understand the other person's perspective on the problem. (3) *List* options for possible plans. (4) *Wait* until they are finished listing before evaluating the options. (5) Talk about *Advantages* and disadvantages of the possible plans (rather than why the other person should be blamed). (6) *Agree* on something, even if it's a minor bit of progress. (7) Be *Polite* to each other throughout.

Anti-Hyperventilation Exercises

Hyperventilation is central to many or perhaps most panic attacks. In the "5 in and 5 out" exercise, the person looks at the stopwatch function of a cell phone or some other display of seconds; they start inhaling when the seconds end in zero and start exhaling when the seconds end in 5. It is very difficult to hyperventilate at this rate; in addition, the practice feels relaxing to many people. The "hold your breath and then cure the high CO2" exercise consists of holding the breath, noticing what air hunger or a high CO_2 state feels like, and curing it by taking a couple of deep breaths as soon as it gets unpleasant. The "hyperventilate and cure the low CO2" exercise consists of breathing fast and deep for 5, 10, or 15 breaths, enough to create a barely noticeable feeling of lightheadedness, and curing that by breathing very slowly, e.g., one respiration over half a minute. The second and third of these exercises are meant to help the brain distinguish accurately between the feelings of too much and too little carbon dioxide, and thus to obviate the error leading to the vicious cycle of hyperventilation.

Breathe and Relax the Muscles

As a preliminary, the person practices tensing and relaxing muscles long enough to learn how to send relaxation signals to every muscle group of the body. When doing this exercise, the person sits comfortably; with every inhalation they get a group of muscles in mind; with every exhalation they relax as much as possible the muscle group selected.

The Loving Kindness Meditation

The person thinks, "May I become the best I can become. May I give and receive kindness. May I live with compassion and peace." Then the person wishes the same things for someone else, and then someone else, and so on. They also might want to wish these things for all humanity.

Decision Practice (SOIL ADDLE)

The person takes a choice point, hypothetical or real, and practices going through steps of decision-making with it. S: They study and describe the *situation* they are in, and search for the most decision-relevant aspects of it. O: They identify their *objectives*. What are they trying to maximize or minimize? I: They seek *information*. What facts will be of aid in making a good decision? L: They *list* options. A: They list the *advantages* and disadvantages of the best options. D: They *decide* upon an option or set of them. D: They *do* what they have decided. LE: They *learn* from the *experience*, while avoiding overgeneralizing.

Social Conversation

While most of us wouldn't consider ordinary social chatting as a "psychological skills exercise," the ability for social conversation to be a "mutually gratifying activity" is a major contributor to positive relationships, which are in turn a major determinant of happiness and mental health (Lemay et al., 2022; Jain, 2023). Accordingly, social chatting should be part of the psychological skills education of every child, whether the learning takes place entirely by incidental, informal learning, or whether it's assisted by more structured means. In psychoeducational tutoring, social conversation can be facilitated by using a list of questions that help in getting to know another person, some sentence-completion exercises, or the "two truths and a lie" game, as supplements to teaching about listening skills as mentioned previously.

7.7 Academic Skills as Psychological Skills

Our culture tends to make a clear divide between such skills as reading, math, and writing, and skills such as conflict-resolution, emotional regulation, decision-making, anger control, choosing self-talk, and so forth. Motor skills such as agility, coordination, endurance, strength, and flexibility are in another sharply demarcated realm. But all of these are skills that make life better, and all of them can be taught by modeling, practice, reinforcement, instruction, and the other influence methods reviewed earlier.

And there is abundant evidence that academic skills are associated with mental health. A study by Stanton (1987) found that the negative relationship between IQ and conduct problems, which has been often found, disappeared when reading skills were partialed out. Morgan et al. (2008) provided evidence that reading difficulties and behavior difficulties cause each other. Pickren et al. (2024) meta-analyzed the correlation between reading and externalizing behavior, reporting a correlation of 0.2 between aggression and teacher ratings of externalizing behavior (where 0.1 and

0.3 are usually taken as thresholds for small and medium effect size for correlations). There is a little research not only documenting correlations, but also that interventions targeting academic skills can enhance mental health variables. Coie and Krehbiel (1984) found that academic skills training actually improved the sociometric status of children more than social skills training did.

7.8 Some Elements of Reading Instruction

In the USA, reading teaching for children of lower socioeconomic status appears to be, on the average, failing. The state of New York ranks first in the USA for dollars spent per child in public education. But according to 2022–2023 test results, only 45% of New York public school third graders scored in the "proficient" level in English language arts, and only 30% of students from low-income backgrounds did so (Education Trust, 2024). Individual tutoring in reading, however, has produced very positive results (Neitzel et al., 2021).

The following are some of the most important concepts of reading instruction, drawn from several decades of carrying out and supervising reading tutoring by Strayhorn (2009).

The most important idea is what we have referred to earlier by the word "hierarchy": the pathway toward learning to read can be delineated as a series of steps, a series of challenges to master. For any given learner at any given time, there is a set of activities that are neither too hard nor too easy, challenging enough to produce progress, at the just right level on the hierarchy for that child. If the tutor can find the right level at any time for the child, not only can this help the rate of progress to be maximized, but even more importantly, it can help to optimize the child's emotional experience in learning. In other words, the learning process can be fun for the child.

We can order stages of reading development as follows:

1. Oral language development. For some children, even of school age, the first priority is tasks that ordinarily are major achievements of the preschool years: enlarging vocabulary and the repertoire of understanding and producing oral language. Reading stories, doing dramatic play, and promoting lots of talk back and forth ("reciprocal interaction") are some of the major activities for development in this realm. Tests of language development help assess how high a priority these skills are.

2 and 3. Phonemic awareness and spatial awareness. These are foundation skills for reading. Phonemic awareness skills include those of hearing separate sounds and blending them to form a word, and hearing a word and segmenting it into separate sounds. Spatial awareness skills include distinguishing right from left, telling whether pairs of images are identical or mirror images, and distinguishing among the lower case letters b, d, p, and q. Some children acquire these skills with no formal teaching before entering school; for others, teaching these skills can provide the missing link whose absence has been frustrating the child daily.

4. Letter-sound correspondence. This is learning a sound for each of the 26 letters—the sounds that the letters make in short, regular, words.

5. Sounding and blending. This is looking at words, saying the sound of each of the letters (or combinations of letters that make a phoneme) and then blending those sounds together to say the word. Words are arranged in order of difficulty, into lists. Within any given list, the words in that list follow the same phonetic principle, so that interference is minimized within that list at least. Sounding and blending exercises each of the three previous skills: phonemic awareness, spatial awareness, and letter-sound correspondence. After sounding and blending the words in a list, sometimes several times, the next step in "word list work" is to read off the words without segmenting the sounds.

6. Text reading: The learner reads a series of texts, with any given text at the correct point on the hierarchy of complexity that the learner is ready for. Instructors may wish to measure the learner's comprehension of what is read, as well as the accuracy.

Although these tasks are presented roughly in order of complexity, several of them can be worked on simultaneously—it is not necessary to finish one before starting another. Within each of these, there is a hierarchy of difficulty just for that stage. Sometimes learners can work at the high end of the hierarchy for one stage while simultaneously working at the low end of the hierarchy for another.

A second principle is that learners vary widely with respect to how much repetitive practice they need with one task in the reading hierarchy before mastery has been achieved. We can think of "reading disability" or "dyslexia" as a condition where the learner needs much more practice to gain the skills than other learners. But if the practice can be made pleasant, the goal can eventually be reached.

A third principle is that the main element that makes repetitive practice pleasant is the enthusiastic positive feedback of a human being with whom the learner has a positive relationship.

A fourth principle is that as soon as the learner can read any text at all, they can read positive models of psychological skills. As they progress, they can read psychological skills instructions and models of higher and higher complexity. But even before they can read text, they can have experiences that strengthen psychological skills through a positive relationship with a tutor and lots of positive reinforcement for productivity and cooperation. Thus, fostering reading and fostering other psychological skills are synergistic goals and are not in competition with one another.

How successful has individual tutoring for reading been? In 1984, Benjamin Bloom wrote of the "2 sigma problem": the search for methods of group instruction as effective as one-to-one tutoring, which according to the work Bloom reviewed, was 2 standard deviations more effective than classroom instruction. The tutoring Bloom referred to combined individual instruction with mastery learning, which can be conceived of as an enlightened use of the principle of hierarchy referred to above. Subsequent studies reviewed in a 2020 meta-analysis (Nickow et al., 2020) found a 0.37 standard deviation effect size for tutoring, which the authors referred to as "impressive," but far from the 2 standard deviations found by Bloom. Strayhorn and Bickel (2003) reported that learners who had prior to tutoring advanced by about 0.5 grade levels per year progressed at 1.5 grade levels per year during tutoring. In this study, tutors kept track of the number of points children achieved in sounding and blending practice (2 points per sound and blend, 1 point for reading the word without segmenting). The point total was strongly related to progress; the regression coefficient indicated that about one grade level of progress was on average associated with every 12,000 points accumulated. (Other activities were also done, so the relationship is not of direct causality.) With about 150 points being a comfortable level of word list work per session, and comparable other activities, e.g., text reading, also done, that would predict one grade level per 80 sessions; at 5 sessions a such progress would be achieved in 16 s. Regarding behavior, the subset of children with ADHD symptoms as rated by teachers at levels compatible with a diagnosis of ADHD were studied. The tutors' ratings of their ADHD and oppositional defiant disorder symptoms were lower than those rated by classroom teachers preintervention, by 2.5 and 1.1 standard deviations, respectively. Teachers' ratings of ADHD symptoms improved significantly over the course of the intervention (effect size 0.9) whereas teachers' ratings of ODD symptoms did not. Strayhorn (2005), reporting on reading tutoring carried out by telephone, reported that a group of learners who had progressed at a rate of 0.44 grade levels per year prior to tutoring progressed at 2.0 grade levels per year during tutoring.

The impression left by research to date is that individual reading tutoring, with careful attention to where the child is at any moment on the hierarchies of difficulty and much joyous reinforcement of the child's productivity, is an intervention with great potential not only for promoting academic skill, but also for promoting mental health.

References

Abramson, L. Y., Seligman, M. E. P., & Teasdale, J. D. (1978). Learned helplessness in humans: Critique and reformulation. *Journal of Abnormal Psychology, 87*(1), 49–74.

Anderson, C. A., Bushman, B. J., Donnerstein, E., Hummer, T. A., & Warburton, W. A. (2017). Screen violence and youth behavior. *Psychological Science in the Public Interest, 18*(1), 1–53. https://doi.org/10.1177/1529100617727680

Bettmann, J. E., Speelman, E., Blumenthal, E., Couch, S., & McArthur, T. (2024). How does nature exposure affect adults with symptoms of mental illness? A meta-analysis. *International Journal of Mental Health Nursing, 33*(6), 1889–1907. https://doi.org/10.1111/inm.13400

Bloom, B. S. (1984). The 2 sigma problem: The search for methods of group instruction as effective as one-to-one tutoring. *Educational Researcher, 13*(6), 4–16.

Burkhouse, K. L., Uhrlass, D. J., Stone, L. B., Knopik, V. S., & Gibb, B. E. (2012). Expressed emotion-criticism and risk of depression onset in children. *Journal Of Clinical Child and Adolescent Psychology, 41*(6), 771–777. https://doi.org/10.1080/15374416.2012.703122

Carpiniello, B. (2023). The mental health costs of armed conflicts—A review of systematic reviews conducted on refugees, asylum-seekers, and people living in war zones. *International Journal of Environmental Research and Public Health, 20*(4), 2840. https://doi.org/10.3390/ijerph20042840

Carvalho, J. P., & Hopko, D. R. (2011). Behavioral theory of depression: Reinforcement, learned helplessness, and beyond. *Psychological Record, 61*(3), 433–451.

Chang, E. C., D'Zurilla, T. J., & Sanna, L. J. (2004). *Social problem solving: Theory, research, and training*. American Psychological Association.

Coie, J. D., & Krehbiel, G. (1984). Effects of academic tutoring on the social status of low-achieving, socially rejected children. *Child Development, 55*, 1465–1478.

Copeland, W. E., Wolke, D., Angold, A., & Costello, E. J. (2013). Adult psychiatric outcomes of bullying and being bullied by peers in childhood and adolescence. *JAMA Psychiatry, 70*(4), 419–426. https://doi.org/10.1001/jamapsychiatry.2013.504

Csikszentmihalyi, M. (1990). *Flow: The psychology of optimal experience*. Harper & Row.

The Education Trust–New York. (2024). *Warning bells: The state of annual 3–8 assessments in New York*. https://newyork.edtrust.org

Eiraldi, R., Power, T. J., Schwartz, B. S., Keiffer, J. N., McCurdy, B. L., Mathen, M., & Jawad, A. F. (2016a). Examining effectiveness of group cognitive-behavioral therapy for externalizing and internalizing disorders in urban schools. *Behavior Modification, 40*(4), 611–639.

Eiraldi, R., Mautone, J. A., Khanna, M. S., & Power, T. J. (2016b). Integrating behavioral health services into pediatric primary care: Improving access and outcomes. *Clinical Psychology: Science and Practice, 23*(4), 372–386.

Frankl, V. E. (2006). *Man's search for meaning* (I. Lasch, Trans.). Beacon Press. (Original work published 1946).

Franklin, B. (1772). Letter to Joseph Priestley, September 19, 1772. In L. W. Labaree et al. (Eds.), *The papers of Benjamin Franklin* (Vol. 19, pp. 299–300). Yale University Press.

Galea, S., Ahern, J., Rudenstine, S., Wallace, Z., & Vlahov, D. (2005). Urban built environment and depression: A multilevel analysis. *Journal of Epidemiology & Community Health, 59*(10), 822–827.

Glick, B., & Gibbs, J. C. (2011). *Aggression replacement training: A comprehensive intervention for aggressive youth* (3rd ed.). Research Press.

Gray, P., Senabe, S., Naicker, N., Kgalamono, S., Yassi, A., & Spiegel, J. M. (2019). Workplace-based organizational interventions promoting mental health and happiness among healthcare workers: A realist review. *International Journal of Environmental Research and Public Health, 16*(22), 4396. https://doi.org/10.3390/ijerph16224396

Haidt, J. (2024). *The anxious generation: How the great rewiring of childhood is causing an epidemic of mental illness*. Penguin Press.

Jackson, D. B., Testa, A., & Vaughn, M. G. (2019). New evidence of the nexus between neighborhood violence, perceptions of danger, and child health. *Health Affairs, 38*(10), 1671–1678. https://doi.org/10.1377/hlthaff.2018.05127

Jain, S. (2023). The association between relationship quality, self-esteem and mental wellbeing in different phases in life from young to middle adulthood. *International Journal of Novel Research and Development, 8*(5), 915–920.

Jimenez, M. P., DeVille, N. V., Elliott, E. G., Schiff, J. E., Wilt, G. E., Hart, J. E., & James, P. (2021). Associations between nature exposure and health: A review of the evidence. *International Journal of Environmental Research and Public Health, 18*(9), 4790. https://doi.org/10.3390/ijerph18094790

Kraav, S. L., Lehto, S. M., Junttila, N., Ruusunen, A., Kauhanen, J., Hantunen, S., & Tolmunen, T. (2021). Depression and loneliness may have a direct connection without mediating factors. *Nordic Journal of Psychiatry, 75*(7), 553–557. https://doi.org/10.1080/08039488.2021.1894231

Leijten, P., Melendez-Torres, G. J., Knerr, W., & Gardner, F. (2016). Transported versus home-grown parenting interventions for reducing disruptive child behavior: A multilevel meta-regression study. *Journal of the American Academy of Child and Adolescent Psychiatry, 55*(7), 610–617. https://doi.org/10.1016/j.jaac.2016.05.003

Leijten, P., Gardner, F., Melendez-Torres, G. J., van Aar, J., Hutchings, J., Schulz, S., Knerr, W., & Overbeek, G. (2019). Meta-analyses: Key parenting program components for disruptive child behavior. *Journal of the American Academy of Child and Adolescent Psychiatry, 58*(2), 180–190. https://doi.org/10.1016/j.jaac.2018.07.900

Lemay, E. P., Le, B. M., & Clark, M. S. (2022). Listening and the pursuit of communal relationships. *Current Opinion in Psychology, 43*, 120–125.

McCartney, G., Hearty, W., Arnot, J., Popham, F., Cumbers, A., & McMaster, R. (2019). Impact of political economy on population health: A systematic review of reviews. *American Journal of Public Health, 109*(6), e1–e12. https://doi.org/10.2105/AJPH.2019.305001

McGee, R. E., & Thompson, N. J. (2015). Unemployment and depression among emerging adults in 12 states: Behavioral risk factor surveillance system, 2010. *Preventing Chronic Disease, 12*, 140451. https://doi.org/10.5888/pcd12.140451

Moore, P., Williams H. J., Evans A. T. (2023). *When mass shooters are seeking fame*. RAND Corporation. https://www.rand.org/pubs/commentary/2023/07/when-mass-shooters-are-seeking-fame.html

Morgan, P. L., Farkas, G., Tufis, P. A., & Sperling, R. A. (2008). Are reading and behavior problems risk factors for each other? *Journal of Learning Disabilities, 41*(5), 417–436. https://doi.org/10.1177/0022219408321123

Morganstein, J. C., Bromet, E. J., & Shigemura, J. (2023). The neuropsychiatric aftermath of exposure to weapons of mass destruction: applying historical lessons to protect health during the war in Ukraine. *Psychological Medicine, 53*(11), 5353–5355. https://doi.org/10.1017/S0033291722002872

National Institute on Drug Abuse. (2018). *Common comorbidities with substance use disorders*. National Institutes of Health, U.S. Department of Health and Human Services. https://www.drugabuse.gov

Neitzel, A. J., Lake, C., Pellegrini, M., Inns, A., & Slavin, R. E. (2021). A synthesis of research on reading interventions for struggling readers in grades K–5. *Reading Research Quarterly, 56*(S1), S229–S250.

Nickow, A., Oreopoulos, P., & Quan, V. (2020). *The impressive effects of tutoring on PreK-12 learning: A systematic review and meta-analysis of the experimental evidence*. National Bureau Of Economic Research (NBER) Working Paper No. 27476, JEL No. I2,J2.

Ogbaselase, F. A., Mancini, K. J., & Luebbe, A. M. (2022). Indirect effect of family climate on adolescent depression through emotion regulatory processes. *Emotion (Washington, D.C.), 22*(5), 1017–1029. https://doi.org/10.1037/emo0000899

Park, C., Majeed, A., Gill, H., Tamura, J., Ho, R. C., Mansur, R. B., Nasri, F., Lee, Y., Rosenblat, J. D., Wong, E., & McIntyre, R. S. (2020). The effect of loneliness on distinct health outcomes: A comprehensive review and meta-analysis. *Psychiatry Research, 294*, 113514. https://doi.org/10.1016/j.psychres.2020.113514

Patterson, G. R. (1975). *Families: Applications of social learning to family life*. Research Press.

Peñuelas, J., & Nogué, S. (2023). Catastrophic climate change and the collapse of human societies. *National Science Review, 10*(6), nwad082.

Pickren, S. E., Torelli, J. N., Miller, A. H., & Chow, J. C. (2024). The relation between reading and externalizing behavior: A correlational meta-analysis. *Annals of Dyslexia, 74*(2), 158–186. https://doi.org/10.1007/s11881-024-00307-w

Rideout, V. J., Foehr, U. G., & Roberts, D. F. (2010). *Generation M^2: Media in the lives of 8- to 18-year-olds. Kaiser Family Foundation*. https://www.kff.org/other/event/generation-m2-media-in-the-lives-of-8-to-18-year-olds/

Rideout, V., & Robb, M. B. (2019). *The Common Sense Census: Media use by tweens and teens*. Common Sense Media. https://www.commonsensemedia.org/research/the-common-sense-census-media-use-by-tweens-and-teens-2019

Rideout, V., Peebles, A., Mann, S., & Robb, M. B. (2022). *The Common Sense Census: Media use by tweens and teens, 2021*. Common Sense Media. https://www.commonsensemedia.org/research/the-common-sense-census-media-use-by-tweens-and-teens-2021

Ridley, M., Rao, G., Schilbach, F., & Patel, V. (2020). Poverty, depression, and anxiety: Causal evidence and mechanisms. *Science, 370*(6522), eaay0214.

Rosenberg, M. B. (2015). *Nonviolent communication: A language of life* (3rd ed.). PuddleDancer Press.

Siegel, M., Ross, C. S., & King, C. (2013). The relationship between gun ownership and firearm homicide rates in the United States, 1981–2010. *American Journal of Public Health, 103*(11), 2098–2105. https://doi.org/10.2105/AJPH.2013.301409

Stanton, W. R. (1987). The relationship between reading ability, intelligence, and behavior problems in children. *Journal of Abnormal Child Psychology, 15*(2), 211–221.

Strayhorn, J. M. (1983). A diagnostic axis relevant to psychotherapy and preventive mental health. *American Journal of Orthopsychiatry, 53*, 677–696.

Strayhorn, J. M. (1988). *The competent child: An approach to psychotherapy and preventive mental health*. Guilford Press.

Strayhorn, J. M. (2001). *Exercises for psychological skills*. Psychological Skills Press.

Strayhorn, J. M. (2005). Pilot study of telephone tutoring in reading skills. *Perceptual and Motor Skills, 101*, 505–509.

Strayhorn, J. M. (2006). *A programmed course in conflict-resolution and anger control: Toward nonviolence and harmony in human relations*. Psychological Skills Press.

Strayhorn, J. M. (2009). *Manual for tutors and teachers of reading* (2nd ed.). Psychological Skills Press.

Strayhorn, J. M. (2013). *A programmed course in psychological skills exercises*. Psychological Skills Press.

Strayhorn, J. M., & Bickel, D. D. (2003). A randomized trial of individual tutoring for elementary school children with reading and behavior difficulties. *Psychological Reports, 92*, 427–444.

Wilkialis, L., Rodrigues, N., Majeed, A., Lee, Y., Lipsitz, O., Gill, H., Tamura, J., Nasri, F., Lui, L. M. W., Siegel, A., Mansur, R. B., Rosenblat, J. D., & McIntyre, R. S. (2021). Loneliness-based impaired reward system pathway: Theoretical and clinical analysis and application. *Psychiatry Research, 298*, 113800. https://doi.org/10.1016/j.psychres.2021.113800

Wolke, D., Copeland, W. E., Angold, A., & Costello, E. J. (2013). Impact of bullying in childhood on adult health, wealth, crime, and social outcomes. *Psychological Science, 24*(10), 1958–1970. https://doi.org/10.1177/0956797613481608

Xu, L., Nan, J., & Lan, Y. (2020). The nucleus accumbens: A common target in the comorbidity of depression and addiction. *Frontiers in Neural Circuits, 14*, 37. https://doi.org/10.3389/fncir.2020.00037

Chapter 8
Evidence So Far on Psychoeducation

Abstract In not-so-ancient times a few decades ago, some serious scholars raised doubts as to whether competences could prevent mental disorder, and as to whether societal factors could cause mental illness. At the time of this writing, the studies on these questions are so numerous as to give rise to a new type of journal article: "umbrella reviews" of systematic reviews and meta-analyses. There is abundant evidence that teaching competences can significantly affect the most prevalent disorders: depression, anxiety, insomnia, substance abuse, aggressive behavior, and relationship difficulties, and even psychotic disorders and bipolar disorder. Competence development has been fostered in settings as disparate as programs training parents to work with their preschool children, self-help groups for adults, self-administered training via Internet or by ordinary books, and importantly, programs for "social and emotional learning" in schools, including those focused on cross-age tutoring. Much modeling, practice opportunities, and reinforcement for maladaptive patterns, delivered through the mass media, are a major obstacle to be overcome. Nonetheless, the demonstration of significant effects with relatively small doses of intervention fosters a vision of what good could be done if society were to really take seriously the delivery of psychoeducation.

Keywords Psychoeducation · Depression · Anxiety · Insomnia · Substance abuse · Parent training · Self-help groups · Bibliotherapy · Online virtual therapy · Media violence · Social and emotional learning · Cross-age tutoring · Psychoeducation for schizophrenia

J. M. Strayhorn, Jr. et al., *The Promise of Psychoeducation in Relieving the Societal Burden of Psychopathology*, SpringerBriefs in Modern Perspectives on Disability Research, https://doi.org/10.1007/978-981-92-0922-4_1

8.1 Can Psychoeducation Prevent or Treat Diagnosable Disorder? Early Criticisms of Prevention, Versus Subsequent Evidence

This book puts forward the idea that biological, learning-based, and environmental influences all contribute to mental health or illness, and that people's learnings can not only improve their own mental health (including reducing diagnosable mental disorder) but also help them to provide more mental-health-friendly environments for others. But this idea has had its critics. Lamb and Zusman (1982) wrote, "Building competence is a worthy goal in and of itself. There is, however, no evidence that it prevents mental disorder." They spoke of "the fundamental flaw of a lack of good evidence for a causal relationship between societal factors and mental illness." These authors quoted favorably from a 1965 book by James Davis: "Mental health educators have little or nothing specific and practical to tell the public" (p. 138). "For instance, even if environmental and situational stresses do play an important role in causing emotional distress, mental health educators still do not possess a body of knowledge that enables them to say anything more than 'Do not be poor or ignorant, and stay out of armed combat'" (p. 139).

As we write, it is now 61 years after Davis's book and 44 years after Lamb and Zusman's chapter. It is safe to say that the claim of "no evidence" that competences can prevent or remediate mental disorders is definitively false (leaving aside the question of whether it was true in the 1960s or 1980s). This chapter will review a tiny portion of the evidence that could be cited.

As a quick start on such evidence: Cognitive behavior therapy is surely a competence-based intervention (the most emphasized competence, but not the only one taught, is that of making good choices about one's own self-talk). There have now been over 2000 outcome studies demonstrating the efficacy of CBT for diagnosable disorders (Beck, 2021, p. 5). Several studies have found that people who have received CBT have continued to improve after therapy termination (von Brachel et al., 2019; Melin et al., 2020). Psychotherapy has had a medium effect size even in people with depression resistant to medications (Ijaz et al., 2020). As a quick comment on the causal relationship between societal factors and mental illness: the fact that post-traumatic stress disorder has been diagnosed in 5% of US adolescents 13–18 years old (Merikangas et al., 2010) seems sufficient, without even referring to a mountain of other evidence, to dispute any claims that environmental and social determinants are inconsequential.

Can the competences needed for societal mental health be imparted by psychoeducation that is potentially, or demonstrably, scalable? This is the more challenging question; the studies cited in this chapter pertain to this. In this chapter, we'll organize partly by diagnosis, since people are so accustomed to dividing up the pie in that way, despite the fact that almost all psychological competences are relevant to more than one official diagnosis. And we'll organize partly by the setting and type of intervention, e.g., parent training or SEL (social and emotional learning, in schools).

We'll focus primarily on the question: To what extent can teaching psychological skills in potentially scalable ways have positive effects? But several other questions underlie, that we won't examine in great detail. If imparting a certain set of skills is effective in remediating a disorder, can we safely infer that the same skills will tend to prevent many cases of it from occurring in the first place? Should psychoeducational interventions be aimed at one particular target, i.e., depression, anxiety, or substance use, or should they teach a broad spectrum of skills, since both skills and diagnoses overlap so much with each other? Since objections have been raised to preventive psychoeducation on the grounds that this may drain funds from those available for treatment, how expensive are various forms of psychoeducation? People's making use of written or video material posted on the Internet can have a marginal cost of zero; one-to-one tutoring in psychological skills can vary depending upon whether the tutors are highly trained professionals or older youth taught to tutor younger ones. And finally, whenever there is a trial of psychoeducation, in what dose is it delivered—how many repetitions of practice, how many hours on task—and what would a dose-response curve look like? More specifically, when positive effects of modest size from modest doses are found, what could be found if the doses of instruction, models, practice, reinforcement, etc. were dramatically raised? As we review research, it's crucial to remember that the effect size reported for a given intervention is just the effect size for whatever *dose* of intervention the researchers chose to study.

8.2 Psychoeducation Aimed at Preventing or Remediating Depression

What do mental health educators have to say to the public that is specific and practical regarding how not to be depressed? A prominent behavioral part of cognitive behavior therapy, i.e., behavior activation therapy, harnesses a simple but powerful idea: figure out things you will either enjoy doing or feel good about having done, get yourself to do them even when you "don't feel like it," and rejoice in having done them. The fundamental idea of cognitive therapy is likewise simple: pay attention to what you say to yourself and imagine, and choose your self-talk and mental imagery so as to help yourself toward your best functioning. Another prominent idea is that increased happiness and less depression are the products of good decisions—of good skills in "social problem-solving." Among these skills are having an orientation toward problem-solving grounded in the beliefs that what one does in problem situations or choice points makes a difference; that one is capable of discriminating better options from worse options; that in important choice points it is better to work toward making a good choice than impulsively to do the first thing that comes to mind or to avoid thinking about the situation; that it is good to be able to discriminate which choices deserve careful thought and which of them are not worth spending much time on. In addition to these attitudes, specific skills of option-generating, evaluating options through consequence-prediction (or generation of pros and cons), and implementing the decisions one has made, can be developed through psychoeducation. Another antidepressant tactic focuses on the fact that happiness and freedom from depression are highly related to the quality of people's relationships, and a number of skills enhance relationships: anger control, kindness, listening skills, social conversation, communicating positive regard, assertion, conflict resolution, cultivating mutually gratifying activities, and others. Physical exercise is now an established antidepressant, and having the self-discipline or resourcefulness to find ways to actually accomplish exercise are skills that can be fostered. Indeed, of 62 psychological skills listed in a previous chapter, it is difficult to find one of them that is not plausibly linked to greater happiness and less depression.

Let's examine a little of the vast amount of evidence regarding the effect of teaching psychological competences upon depression.

We'll start with bibliotherapy—just giving people curated information to read—because this is obviously scalable, cheap, and not psychotherapy. Its effects were initially studied as a control intervention compared to active treatment, but when evidence emerged that it could be effective for mild to moderate depression, it became an intervention of interest in and of itself (Cuijpers, 1997, p. 140). Bibliotherapy is a subset of self-help; while inspiration and information can be drawn from a wide variety of materials such as books, autobiographies, internet materials, films, and support groups (Norcross, 2006), bibliotherapy is specifically intended to be independently learned and applied (McKendree-Smith et al., 2003) with no or minimal supportive guidance from a professional or paraprofessional. It may take the form of "written texts, computer programs or audio/video-recorded material for the purpose of understanding or solving problems concerning a person's development or in meeting their therapeutic needs" (Marrs 1995, as cited in den Boer, 2004).

Usually, bibliotherapy draws from cognitive-behavioral psychotherapies, because they are more psychoeducational in nature and hence more appropriate for self-administration, unlike, for example, psychodynamic and experiential psychotherapies (McKendree-Smith et al., 2003, p. 283). Two examples of prominent bibliotherapy resources, i.e., David Burns' *Feeling Good* (1980), and Peter Lewinsohn's *Control Your Depression* (1986), have also been featured in several studies of cognitive bibliotherapy, with quite a number of studies showing positive results.

In a population of depressed older adults, Scogin et al. (1987) compared bibliotherapy using *Feeling Good* to a book less directly related to depression (Frankl's *Man's Search for Meaning*) and a waitlist control. The cognitive bibliotherapy group improved more than the other two conditions. Follow-up showed that gains were maintained at 6 months and 2 years after, despite the fact that most of them had not received any additional treatment (Scogin et al., 1990). In another study with depressed older adults, Scogin et al. (1989) compared bibliotherapy using *Feeling Good*, with behavioral bibliotherapy using Lewinsohn's *Control Your Depression*, and a waitlist control. Results indicated that both bibliotherapy groups improved significantly and maintained gains at 2-year follow-up, and neither bibliotherapy condition was superior to the other. Some newer studies have also replicated these findings. Floyd et al. (2004) compared cognitive bibliotherapy to 16 sessions of individual cognitive psychotherapy for depression in older adults. Participants in both cognitive bibliotherapy and individual cognitive therapy did better at posttreatment than the waiting conditions, with cognitive therapy showing only a slight advantage that disappeared at 3-month follow-up as bibliotherapy participants continued to improve. Floyd et al. (2006) further found that in both the therapy and bibliotherapy conditions, progress was maintained at 2-year follow-up. In the general adult population, Jamison and Scogin (1995) found bibliotherapy using *Feeling Good* to be efficacious in reducing depression as compared to a waitlist control. In addition, the treatment group kept their gains 3 months following treatment, and the waitlist control participants also improved posttreatment. Gains were also found to be maintained at 3-year follow-up (Smith et al., 1997). Among adolescents with mild to moderate depression, cognitive bibliotherapy has also been found to be superior to delayed-treatment control in reducing depression and depressogenic attitudes, and participants continued to improve at 1-month follow-up (Ackerson et al., 1998).

Not all trials of bibliotherapy have proclaimed victories. A study by Joling et al. (2011) found bibliotherapy no better than usual care for depression; authors saw low motivation in the sample as the reason for lack of effect. Naylor et al. (2010) found bibliotherapy no more effective than treatment as usual, where treatment as usual included exercise, increased clinician attention, and medication. Mead et al. (2005) found no evidence for superiority of bibliotherapy over wait list control. As with all psychoeducation (and psychotherapy), the degree of effort put into the mission by the participants can vary widely and has obvious relation to efficacy. In the Naylor et al. (2010) study, the total number of pages read by the participants varied widely and were mostly well under a quarter of the pages assigned. There was no significant correlation between the number of pages completed and the final depression score.

Overall, the effect size of cognitive bibliotherapy for depression has emerged in several meta-analyses as large: 0.77 in one (Gregory et al., 2004, 17 studies), and 0.80 in another (Gellatly et al., 2007, 34 studies), and 0.84 at posttreatment and 0.76 at follow-up (den Boer et al., 2004, 14 studies). Anderson et al. (2005, 6 studies) reported an effect size of −1.36 (negative better) in a meta-analysis of the effects of *Feeling Good* compared with delayed treatment. A review by Gualano et al. (2017) reported that in adults, bibliotherapy was found superior to no treatment and non-inferior to treatment with medication. Bibliotherapy was less effective with children and adolescents in studies reviewed by Gualano et al. (2017). Gellatly and colleagues found that self-help may be more effective in the form of treatment rather than of preventive care, and cognitive-behavioral techniques were more effective than simple educational material. Furthermore, they noted that facilitation by a professional or paraprofessional who provided support or guidance emerged as a significant moderating factor; however, this has also been contradicted elsewhere (Gregory et al., 2004).

Bibliotherapy in schools is a logical way to simultaneously promote academic and psychological skill. A meta-analysis of bibliotherapy for depression and anxiety in children and adolescents (Yuan et al., 2018) reported a 0.78 effect size for depression outcomes, and 0.36 for anxiety.

Turning from bibliotherapy but staying in the camp of didactic intervention: A much-studied intervention for depression is the *Coping with Depression Course*, developed by Lewinsohn et al. (1984). The subtitle for the manual includes the phrase "psychoeducational intervention." Cuijpers (1998) remarked that in this course, "There is no traditional therapeutic relationship between group leaders and participants. Group leaders are defined as teachers and the participants as pupils" (p. 522). The course is oriented toward increasing the rate of positive reinforcement one receives, and covers several psychological skills: behavioral activation; assertiveness; nonverbal communication; cognitive restructuring; relaxation training; breathing training; problem-solving, including option-generating and evaluating; strengthening supportive relationships; sleep hygiene; exercise; nutrition; and substance abuse awareness. The meta-analysis by Cuijpers (1998) reported a mean effect size of 0.65 for treatment versus control, and 1.21 for pre-to-post change. An adolescent version of the course has been tested, with significant results and gains maintained at 2-year follow-up (Lewinsohn, 1986). A randomized trial of the adolescent version of the *Coping With Depression Course* proved effective even in depressed adolescents with comorbid conduct disorder (Rohde et al., 2004).

Another widely tested program, aimed more at prevention of depression than remediation, is the Penn Resilience Program. Part of this is Martin Seligman's (1998) conceptualization of optimism versus pessimism as determined by whether positive and negative events are viewed as personalized, pervasive, and permanent. Optimistic individuals tend to perceive positive outcomes personalized (that is, a result of their own actions); pervasive (that is, generalized to other situations); and permanent (that is, likely to last). Optimists also tend to attribute the opposite conditions to negative events. Pessimistic individuals tend to have the reverse attributions. The Penn Resilience Program teaches not just the attributions determining optimism versus pessimism, but a variety of other skills having to do with sleep, nutrition, exercise, connecting with others, and having a set of values (University of Pennsylvania, 2026). At least one iteration of the program is delivered by classroom teachers in 18 1-h sessions (Foundations, 2025). A meta-analysis of 17 controlled evaluations of this program (Brunwasser et al., 2009) found significant effect sizes for the program versus no treatment, for depressive symptom score, ranging from 0.11 to 0.21. Effect sizes are almost always lower for preventive programs than for remedial programs, because the presence of people in both groups who would do OK with or without the preventive intervention dilutes effect sizes. As reported with several other psychoeducational interventions, effects appeared to increase during the time from post-intervention to follow-up. But there were no significant differences between outcomes for this program and those for active treatment control conditions. And the program did not reduce the risk for diagnosable depressive disorders, during the time of follow-up.

8.3 Psychoeducation for Anxiety

The field of anxiety reduction is another where there is very strong evidence against the "straw man" argument of "nothing to teach the public" quoted at the beginning of this chapter. Programs for the remediation and prevention of anxiety disorders tend to include various common components. Among these are understanding the manifestations of anxiety, including the flight-or-fight response; understanding the difference between useful or life-saving fear and "false alarms" that interfere with functioning; learning the role of escape and avoidance in maintaining unwanted fears; learning relaxation skills; learning anti-hyperventilation strategies; identifying triggers for unwanted fear and ordering situations in a hierarchy according to how much fear they elicit; becoming aware of and practicing with the types of thoughts that increase and decrease anxiety; starting low on the hierarchy and working the way up, practicing desirable handlings of the trigger situations, in either fantasy rehearsal, real-life exposure, or both; designing self-reinforcement for bits of progress; learning problem-solving skills, including option-generation; and promoting differential reinforcement by family members that favors good functioning over impairment.

The use of such components in traditional cognitive behavior therapy has been shown effective in numerous trials. For example, with social anxiety disorder, Kindred et al. (2022) meta-analyzed 25 studies of CBT and reported posttreatment effect sizes of 0.74 for social anxiety and 0.69 for general anxiety; moreover, upon follow-up 12 months or more after treatment end, symptoms of social anxiety had continued to improve. This study also reported an effect size of 0.52 for depression; it's one of several studies finding that the same intervention was effective for both anxiety and depression.

Lewis et al. (2012) reviewed self-help interventions for anxiety, imposing a 1-h limit upon the time a professional devoted to the learner throughout the entire intervention. Thirty-one randomized clinical trials were found. An effect size of 0.84 relative to waiting list controls was found for the self-help interventions, although the therapist-guided interventions did even better, with a 0.34 difference when the two were compared.

Having outlined mainstream approaches to anxiety in the first paragraph in this section, we should note a very different approach: "Positive Affect Treatment" (Craske et al., 2019, 2022, 2023; Meuret et al., 2022). Rather than attempting to identify situational triggers to fear or aversion and alter the response to those situations, this treatment method seeks only to bring out more experiences of positive affect, and in outcome studies, therapists and clients were explicitly enjoined not to address the negative feelings and the situations that provoke them. The intervention falls clearly into the camp of psychoeducation, despite being delivered one-to-one by therapists, because there was a standard curriculum delivered to all participants, with a workbook and with written assignments to be completed daily. Components of the intervention included furnishing a listing of words for positive emotions, eliciting any memories of when those were experienced, planning activities designed to bring these out, as in Behavior Activation Therapy; and doing a number of exercises meant to increase positive emotion. Examples of the exercises include "silver lining," wherein the learner seeks and finds the positive aspect of a potentially negative or neutral situation; "taking ownership," or recalling positive situations and identifying one's own contributions to a positive outcome (similar to what has been called the "celebrations exercise"); "gratitude," or being aware of blessings bestowed by others or by fate; "generosity," or seeking and finding opportunities to make others happy; "loving-kindness," a meditative technique taken from Buddhist teachings wherein one wishes standard positive outcomes for oneself, for one person after another, and perhaps for all humanity; "appreciative joy," where one identifies good things that have happened to other people and practices deliberately taking pleasure in such (as contrasted with feeling jealous or angry). Craske et al. (2019), in a randomized study, found that positive affect treatment, as compared with more traditional negative affect oriented treatment, yielded, at 6-month follow-up, significantly better outcomes for positive affect, depression, anxiety, stress, and suicidal ideation. Regarding time on task: participants in Positive Affect Treatment were asked to do worksheets daily for 15 weeks.

Turning to anti-anxiety programs for children: The manualized "Coping Cat" program, developed and refined by Philip Kendall and colleagues, and delivering most if not all of the components listed in the first paragraph of this section, has been used in traditional one-to-one cognitive behavior therapy for anxiety in children and youth, but has also been adapted for other settings, included computer-assisted versions (Norris & Kendall, 2020). The Coping Cat model was delivered by individual CBT, and compared with a computer-assisted version (called Camp Cope-a-Lot) administered individually by relatively untrained facilitators, and a support and attention control condition. Rates at which children no longer met criteria for their anxiety diagnosis for the three interventions, respectively, were 70%, 81%, and 19% (Khanna & Kendall, 2010). The computer-assisted version is promising for scalability.

A CBT-based prevention program called FRIENDS was implemented in schools with 9- and 10-year-old children (Stallard et al., 2014). This program, which showed evidence of effectiveness in prior studies (Stallard et al., 2005, 2008), teaches skills that decrease both anxiety and depression and increase resilience. This intervention was carried out in nine 60-min sessions delivered to whole classrooms of children; "usual school provision" classrooms were controls. The intervention, as delivered by trained health professionals, showed a significant, although not huge, improvement in child rated RCADS (Revised Child Anxiety and Depression Scale) scores as compared with usual provision, but the same curriculum as delivered by classroom teachers did not. This study reminds us that as much as we would like psychosocial outcome studies to yield generalizable statements of the form, "This intervention is effective for X outcome with Y effect size," generalizability is elusive. Each particular study's outcome is dependent upon who is delivering it, how they deliver it, who is receiving it, whatever else is going on in the participants' environments, how long the intervention was delivered, how many rehearsals of adaptive skills took place, whether the participants actually wanted to learn the skills taught, whether they worked at the skills or paid attention to them at all, and other factors. This study also provides another example of an intervention where the total intervention time (9 h), for many children, is less than that spent in a few days of playing shooter video games (to be discussed later). But, as with many other psychoeducational interventions, it's reasonable to ask: "If a significant, though modest, effect can be demonstrated with 9 hours of intervention, what would be accomplished by treating mental health skills like math or language arts skills, spending time on them every school day for years?"

8.4 Psychoeducation for Insomnia

Cognitive behavior therapy for insomnia, or CBT-I, consists largely of teaching clients how to improve sleep. What is taught? Clients, or students, are given three central recommendations or directives: (1) Set up a conditioned association between the bed and sleep—by not using the bed for watching TV, using the phone, reading, doing homework, or other activities other than sleep (and sexual activity). Get out of bed and do something non-exciting if one is lying awake unpleasantly. Go to sleep under the same conditions under which one will go back to sleep after an awakening during the night. (2) Increase the association between being in bed and sleeping, by restricting the number of hours in bed to the amount that sleep diaries reveal one is actually spending asleep, or 5 h, whichever is more. Gradually increase the amount of time in bed when the habit of falling asleep upon going to bed is established. (3) Notice any thoughts about how awful or catastrophic it will be if one does not fall asleep, and revise those. Other elements taught may often include the following: (4) Maintain a steady sleep rhythm, particularly keeping constant the time of awakening. Use resetters of the circadian clock, i.e., bright light, exercise, eating, and being out of bed, if one needs to reset the circadian rhythm. (5) Titrate the dose of exercise during the day to the point where physical fatigue helps with sleep. (6) Learn relaxation strategies, for example muscle relaxation. (7) Avoid caffeine, screens, strenuous exercise, and attempts at difficult conflict resolution too close to bedtime. (8) Write, during the daytime, about the to-do list and decisions to be made, as an alternative to going over these while lying in bed. (9) Restrict media exposure, especially those of violent images. (10) Avoid, if possible, any drugs which can interfere with sleep, either by their primary effects or their withdrawal effects.

This sounds like straight instruction. Where does the "therapy" come in? Ideally, the therapist expertly uses the methods of influence reviewed in the previous chapter. The therapist might help the person get motivated and energized to undertake the recommended actions (objective-formation). They might figure out a series of steps toward all these, if the client is overwhelmed at the prospect of doing all this at once (hierarchy). They should nurture rapport (relationship), partly by being an empathic listener. They attribute to the client the ability to succeed (attribution), monitor the client's progress (monitoring), and celebrate with the client each bit of progress (reinforcement). These are not only the methods used by good psychotherapists, but also by good teachers, work supervisors, parents, relationship partners, and others.

How effective is CBT-I? A meta-analysis by Palagini et al. (2024) of CBT-I for adults reported that for insomnia, four out of five studies reviewed reported large effect sizes, i.e., standardized mean differences of 0.8 or larger. Moreover, according to this meta-analysis, targeting sleep remedied depression: there was an average medium effect size (standardized mean difference) of 0.5 for the effect of CBT-I for depression. Mei et al. (2024) meta-analyzed studies of CBT-I for adolescents. Large effect sizes were found for insomnia and sleep-onset latency, and medium effect sizes for total sleep time and sleep efficiency. CBT-I appears better for sleep than melatonin, which is very widely used as a sleep aid. A survey in the USA (American Academy of Sleep Medicine, 2023) found that 29% of respondents reported taking melatonin occasionally or regularly. A meta-analysis by Ferracioli-Oda et al. (2013) reported, with melatonin, an average increase in sleep time of 8.25 min and a decrease in sleep latency of 7.06 min.

The research on CBT-I brings out a semantic problem with the word *psychoeducation*. Another meta-analysis, by Furukawa et al. (2024), states that the most efficacious combination of CBT-I components, when compared with "in-person psychoeducation," seemed to produce a 33% higher rate of remission from insomnia. But CBT-I itself can be thought of as "in-person-psychoeducation." The average control group intervention appeared to consist of psychoeducation carried out with less energy, with less content, or without as strong incentives for the learners to actually master it—in other words, with less well-done psychoeducation. This reminds us that the words we use to report research results usually give the false impression that "intervention labeled x" in one implementation is the same as that bearing the same label in another.

Nonetheless, the data on CBT-I give compelling evidence of effectiveness, with the result that the American College of Physicians' guideline was that adults with chronic insomnia all get CBT-I—and not sleeping pills—as the initial treatment (Qaseem, et al., 2016).

CBT-I as delivered by a licensed professional is not particularly more scalable than other psychotherapy. What evidence is there that the psychoeducation therein can be delivered in less labor-intensive, more scalable forms? A web-based application called Sleepio carries out CBT-I via an animated therapist. Favorable results have been reported for people with chronic insomnia (Espie et al., 2012). Significant effects of CBT-I versus a placebo intervention and "treatment as usual" were reported for a number of variables. Some of the variables studied were sleep efficiency, sleep-onset latency, wake time after sleep onset, impact on daytime performance, impact on social functioning, and total sleep time. A trial of the same intervention with pregnant women with insomnia reported a large effect size difference (Cohen's $d = 1.03$) from treatment as usual (Felder et al., 2020). Another Internet-administered CBT-I program called SHUTi (Sleep Healthy Using The Internet) also reported large effect sizes, also delivering services with "no clinical support"—at least not by humans (Ritterband et al., 2016).

A conclusion from the CBT-I literature to date is that there is a body of information, habits, and skills that is clearly useful in attaining better sleep; imparting all that in a scalable way appears definitely possible, with at least some segments of the population. Efforts to deliver psychoeducation in creative and scalable ways appear quite promising.

8.5 Psychoeducation for Aggression

With civilization facing the possibility of nuclear war; with the most pernicious causes of trauma being people's cruelty to one another; with large fractions of people afraid of walking alone, in the USA at least, for fear of violent attack; with hostile and verbally abusive emotional climates demonstrably causative of psychopathology in adults; with child abuse and adverse childhood experiences of mistreatment generating a wide variety of pathologies; with war veterans having higher rates of suicide than nonveterans; with very significant fractions of children and adolescents being involved in bullying; and with long-term negative consequences on mental health, surely prevention of aggression, violence, cruelty, and the consequences of unbridled anger should be top priority for psychoeducation.

In contrast to our "straw man" claim that mental health educators have little or nothing useful to tell the public, there is hardly a skill listed in Chap. 7 that is *not* relevant to the problem of aggression. If we were to launch into the psychological skill groups enumerated there, we might start by citing that with respect to productivity skills, a study by Nordin and Almén (2017) shows a "strong association between long-term unemployment and violent crime"; with respect to joyousness, Fazel et al. (2015) found that the odds of violent crime were three times higher with depressed than with non-depressed individuals. Learning to turn down flight-or-fight response by relaxation strategies, to use conflict-resolution tactics, to make careful decisions rather than acting on impulse, to develop friendships with favorable emotional climates, to be able to translate verbally abusive utterances to tactful messages, to use fortitude and self-discipline when frustrated, to value kindness and adopt the goal of contributing to other people's happiness, to use fantasy rehearsal to practice difficult acts of anger control, and to have a strong commitment to the ideal of a nonviolent society, all of these should be imparted to humanity with all the resources we can muster.

Let's review some of the psychoeducational interventions that have appeared useful in reducing anger and aggression. Raymond Novaco (Taylor & Novaco, 2022) and Donald Meichenbaum (2001) have been pioneers in the application of cognitive behavior therapy methods to problems of anger and aggression. Elements of such treatment programs have included promoting motivation for change, forming a hierarchy of provocation situations, teaching thought revision regarding provocations, training in lowering physiological arousal, teaching assertiveness and problem-solving skills as an alternative to aggression, and promoting much practice through fantasy rehearsal or role-playing of rational responses to provocations.

Such interventions have been manualized and structured, so as to fall clearly into the camp of psychoeducation: for example, Taylor and Novaco (2022) outline, session by session, the content of a curriculum with 18 sessions, 1 h each. Although intellectual disability is a risk factor for aggression and is often thought of as an impediment to cognitive behavior therapy, Taylor and Novaco reviewed 13 controlled studies of anger control therapy with intellectually disabled samples, 12 of which reported some significant positive outcomes, mostly by participant self-report. Meichenbaum (2001) reviewed and referenced many positive outcome studies for the CBT package called Stress Inoculation Training for anger control. A 2003 meta-analysis by DiGiuseppe and Tafrate for anger control treatment interventions reported moderate and significant levels of improvement relative to control groups and large improvements relative to pre-intervention status. By 2018, enough studies had accumulated for Lee and DiGiuseppe (2018) to review 13 meta-analyses of studies targeting anger and 8 meta-analyses of those targeting aggressive behavior. Six of 13 meta-analyses regarding anger reported average effect sizes of 0.7 standard deviations difference or greater; 4 of 7 regarding aggressive behavior reported average effect sizes of 0.5 or greater.

Aggression Replacement Training is a psychoeducational system based in social learning theory, divisible into three components: anger control (the emotional part), social skills training (the behavior part), and moral reasoning (the values part) (Goldstein et al., 1998; Glick & Gibbs, 2011). Fifty skills are included in the curriculum, including social skills such as introducing yourself, saying thank you, giving a compliment, apologizing, and persuading others; skills regarding emotions such as awareness of one's own feelings, reading cues for others' feelings, and self-reinforcement; and skills for non-aggressive options such as negotiating, assertiveness, and handling teasing. The training is typically given in 3 weekly 90-min sessions per week over 10 weeks. Studies on Aggression Replacement Training exemplify the futility of seeking a single answer to the question, "What is the effect size of this intervention?" If one wants to produce a large effect size, a way to do it is to select motivated and fairly high functioning research participants and measure outcomes by self-reports of anger and aggression. If one wants to take on a challenge that is dramatically more difficult, one delivers the intervention by court order to participants who have been convicted of violent criminal acts, and uses recidivism as the outcome measure. Aggression Replacement Training has taken on some of the biggest challenges (Hornsveld et al., 2015; Smeijers et al., 2018; Kaya & Buzlu, 2016), with some significant positive results, e.g., a 1.08 pre-post effect size in the Smeijers et al. study. Despite this, no studies with violent criminals that we are aware of has claimed anything close to a high "cure rate."

Relaxation training, whether or not aided by biofeedback, is a logical component of anger control programs: training can directly lower the "flight-or-fight" physiology. Positive results have been reported for EMG biofeedback (Kaur & Kaur, 2021), relaxation training (Lopata, 2003), and mindfulness training (O'Dean et al., 2025).

The ideas and instructions of Dialectical Behavior Therapy were first developed as a treatment for Borderline Personality Disorder, for which alternatives to unbridled anger and aggression are major goals; DBT ideas unsurprisingly have been packaged into psychoeducational interventions with relevance to anger and aggression (Chapman & Gratz, 2015). The "problem-solving skill" and the "DEAR MAN" (Describe, Express, Assert, Reinforce…) skills of DBT outline rational conflict resolution strategies. The "opposite action" skill teaches kindness or walking away as alternatives to aggressive behavior. The "STOP" skill (Stop yourself from impulsive action, Take a step back, Observe what is happening, Proceed with the action predicted to produce the best results) is an alternative to impulsive aggression. The "TIPS" skill (Temperature, Intense exercise, Paced breathing, Self-Soothing) provides options for handling intense emotion. Hasselle et al. (2025) meta-analyzed 27 studies using DBT training as a universal, school (including college)-based social and emotional learning program; results were mixed but generally positive, on outcomes including emotional regulation.

The ideal intervention for aggressive behavior does not wait for bad outcomes, but prevents them. Parent training is an intervention very strongly supported by research, particularly for the prevention and remediation of oppositional, conduct, and aggressive problems in children. As with other areas of psychoeducation, the theories behind the teachings are mostly very simple. One central idea is of reinforcement: that behaviors are strongly influenced by their consequences—Thorndike's law of effect, or Skinner's operant learning. This idea was translated to practical parenting by Gerald Patterson and colleagues, beginning in the late 1950s. Reinforcement principles teach parents how to conceptualize, for example, a very common interaction pattern: A child wants something, and the parent says no. After a few unpleasant interchanges between parent and child, the child starts tantruming, throwing things, or hitting. The parent decides that enforcing the command isn't worth the trouble, and with an exasperated "OK, fine!" gives the child what he wanted. The child ceases the unpleasant behavior. The parent's strategy "worked" in the short run to end the tantrum, but it unfortunately increased the probability of future tantrums. The child has now been reinforced for the unpleasant behavior by getting what he wanted, and the parent has been reinforced for giving in to the child by the cessation of the tantrum (this is negative reinforcement). If parents can learn to avoid this common cycle, that in itself is worth the price of admission to parent training. Another parenting pearl is that attention and excitement are often reinforcing for a child, even when the emotional valence of the attention is negative. Thus, the more parents can ignore unwanted behavior and give enthusiastic attention to the positive, i.e., use differential reinforcement in the healthy direction, the more the positive behaviors tend to come out. Patterson (1982) demonstrated another important principle: giving a child lots of commands, particularly in a harsh and critical tone of voice, tends to increase noncompliance by the child. Many parents can greatly benefit from learning to ration commands and to clearly distinguish between commands and suggestions—and to watch and see whether the child complies with each command, and strongly consider saying "thank you" in response to compliance. The art of reflective listening, creation of a positive emotional climate, seeking mutually gratifying activities to do with the child, avoiding violence or threats of it, using time out and/or response cost as consequences for misbehavior where ignoring isn't appropriate, using rational problem-solving conversations (e.g., the Dr.

L.W. Aap strategy described earlier in this book) as an alternative to angry altercations, furnishing positive models for the child both in real life and in fiction and minimizing the exposure to negative models, and setting up programs for tangible reinforcement as well as social reinforcement, when indicated all have been parts of parenting curricula.

As early as 1997, Kazdin summarized "scores" of randomized trials of parent training, with the following conclusions. First, parent training has led to "marked improvements" not only according to parent ratings, but also to ratings by teachers and frequencies of truancy, police contacts, and institutionalization. Parent training has been known to reduce levels of conduct problems to those of normally functioning peers. Treatment gains have been maintained in follow-ups 1 to 3 years after treatment end, and in the case of one study, 10 to 14 years later. There have also been reported improvements in maternal depression and the behavior of siblings. A 2013 Cochrane review (Furlong et al., 2013) reported statistically significant improvements from parent training programs on child conduct problems, parental mental health, parenting skills, and harsh parenting practices. This review reported that "there was a cost of approximately $2500 … per family to bring the average child with clinical levels of conduct problems into the non-clinical range."

One widely tested parenting program is known as The Incredible Years. Webster-Stratton (1998) reported on a randomized trial with 394 Head Start mothers. The intervention resulted in mothers using fewer commands and criticisms and more positivity; children showed fewer conduct problems, less noncompliance, more positive affect and less negative affect, and greater social competence. Treatment gains were mostly maintained a year after training. Another randomized controlled trial of the same curriculum with 634 families (Reid et al., 2001) produced similar results. The sample for this study contained significant fractions of Caucasian, African American, Asian, and Hispanic families, with insignificant differences in treatment response and satisfaction with the intervention among these groups.

Another widely adopted program is the Triple P, Positive Parenting Program, another intellectual descendant of social learning theorists and practitioners. A 2008 meta-analysis by de Graaf et al. found the program effective in reducing disruptive behaviors in children with behavior problems in several settings, particularly with parents with pre-intervention parenting difficulties. Improvements were maintained, with further improvement occurring during the time to follow-up. The overall effect size for pre-intervention versus the 6- or 12-month follow-up, on scores on the Eyberg Child Behavior Inventory, was reported as 1.0. This was larger than the effect at posttreatment, which was 0.88. This is one of several studies where improvement from psychoeducation appears to continue after intervention ends, as contrasted with withdrawal effects. A randomized trial of Triple P delivered online reported improvements in children's problem behavior, and the confidence, anger, and parenting styles of parents. At the 6-month follow-up, gains were maintained, and for some variables, gains were enhanced (Sanders et al., 2012). Day and Sanders (2018) tested Triple P online, delivered in a self-directed way versus with "minimal support" from telephone contacts with practitioners. The self-directed version appeared effective in improving behaviors of both parents and children, but the practitioner-supported version was significantly more effective. It appears that both the self-directed and the practitioner-supported versions are quite scalable.

Parent Management Training, Oregon model, is the program evolved over decades by Patterson and colleagues. Rather than attempting to comprehensively review the many outcome studies of such training, a particular outcome study conducted by this group is instructive. Forgatch and DeGarmo (1999) reported on a randomized trial of parent training with a group of mothers of high-risk background who had recently been divorced, and study of the effects on their sons. Improvements in parenting correlated with improvements in child behavior by parent, child, and teacher report. Follow-up 9 years after intervention revealed not only fewer arrests for the sons of the intervention group than of the control group, but also fewer arrests for the mothers, and better economic conditions for the mothers (Forgatch et al., 2009; Patterson et al., 2010; Laura and John Arnold Foundation, 2017)! Lest we give the impression that the problem of antisocial behavior has been solved by this, the arrest rate in the intervention group was still high enough to be very problematic—about 0.76 arrests per boy—even though it was a little over half the rate for the comparison group (1.34 arrests per boy).

Kazdin et al. (1992) studied parent management training, problem-solving training for children, and both of the above, for the treatment of children with severe antisocial behavior. (There was no group who received neither treatment.) Results confirmed expectations that the combination of teaching both parents and children, parenting and problem-solving, respectively, produced more positive change than either intervention separately.

Enough research on parenting programs had accumulated by 2011 for Bonin et al. (2011) to conclude that the savings to society brought about over 25 years by reduced conduct problems resulting from evidence-based parenting training were about 8 to 17 times higher than the cost of intervention.

The Good Behavior Game is another intervention based on reinforcement principles. It is a school-based intervention in which classes of students are divided into three teams, balanced with regard to their behavior ratings. Teachers communicate the classroom rules. During game periods, teachers keep track of infractions of rules among team members; all teams receive a reward if the team committed four or fewer infractions during the period. Thus, the game rewards students for the absence of aggressive and disruptive behavior, and encourages peers to reinforce each other for the same. The applied behavior analysts refer to this as DRO, differential reinforcement of other (than the undesired behavior), and an interdependent group contingency. In the original intervention, which took place in the 1980s (Kellam et al., 2014), the game periods started at 10 min each and progressed to 25 min for first graders and 40 min for second graders; it was conducted three times a week. Thus, unlike some other interventions, the total number of intervention hours that children experienced probably exceeded 100. In the service of generalization, after the children were used to the game, the teachers would start it without announcing it, and during various activities rather than at a fixed time. Children experienced this during their first and second grades of school, and outcomes were studied over years thereafter. Males identified as highly aggressive in the first 2 years of school and in the control classrooms were reported as having a 100% rate of antisocial personality disorder characteristics around age 19, whereas the rate was 40% for those in the Good Behavior Game classrooms (Kellam et al., 2011). For the same highly aggressive males, the Good Behavior Game appeared to lower the rate of violent and criminal behavior in early adulthood from 50% in control classroom alumni to 34% in Good Behavior Game alumni. These results are at the same time extremely impressive, and also a reminder (as if one were needed) that the problem of antisocial and aggressive behavior is far from solved and probably will not be by any one time-limited intervention. A "third generation" iteration of the Good Behavior Game (Wilcox et al., 2022), which expanded intervention targets, reported positive effects on aggressive behavior. More will be said on the Good Behavior Game in the section on prevention of substance abuse.

A very important approach to prevention of aggression is social and emotional learning programs in schools that include components on kindness, empathy, thinking before acting, generating options when problem-solving, and others. We will discuss these in a section devoted to social and emotional learning.

8.6 Psychoeducation to Prevent Substance Use Disorders

A variety of psychoeducational components are included in nearly every program of remediation of substance abuse problems. In order to keep this section to a reasonable length, we'll look at programs meant to be universal, scalable, and preventive; these have been carried out in schools.

The story of anti-substance-use education provides a cautionary tale, lest we forget that not all education is effective. The largest of such efforts has been Project DARE (Drug Abuse Resistance Education), formed in 1983 by a partnership of the police department and the school district of Los Angeles. Police officers went to schools to deliver mainly lecture-based instruction about the dangers of drugs along with some role-playing of refusal skills. The project grew quickly. The 2002 tax return for the organization reported about $9 million in expenditures by the organization, but efforts by police officers and volunteers were estimated at about $208 million. This tax return stated that the programs were used in 80% of the USA school districts, reaching 26 million students. But as evaluations of the effectiveness of the program came in, the results were not encouraging. They were meta-analyzed in 1994 by Ennett et al., and in 2004 by West and O'Neal. The latter meta-analysis reported a 95% confidence interval for the Cohen's d effect size of the program, as −0.04 to 0.08. Thus, not only did these results fail to reject the null hypothesis; they supported a large degree of confidence that the effects did not come close to reaching what is commonly thought of as a small effect size, i.e., 0.20.

DARE was one component of California's DATE (Drug, Alcohol, and Tobacco Education) program. Other components included education in health and science courses, anti-drug assemblies, "Red Ribbon Weeks," and counseling. Brown et al. (1995) interviewed or surveyed over 5000 student recipients of such education;

39.4% of the respondents reported a neutral feeling about those who delivered the education, and 30% reported a negative emotional response. Ninety percent of high schoolers communicated a preference for information delivered in some other way.

Perhaps in response to findings of low effectiveness, the DARE curriculum has been revised; the new version is labeled Keepin' it REAL. (REAL is an acronym for ways of turning down an offer of a drug: Refuse, Explain, Avoid, Leave.) A study of the revised curriculum with fifth grade students reported statistically significant results in students receiving the curriculum with respect to alcohol use, drunkenness, and vaping, when compared to virtual controls. The incidence of these behaviors in the sample was "extremely low," and thus the effect sizes appear to be small, although they are not reported directly in the study (Hansen et al., 2023). A translation of the DARE Keepin' it REAL curriculum into Portuguese has been widely implemented in Brazil. A randomized trial of this curriculum, compared to no intervention, for fifth graders in 28 schools and seventh graders in 30 schools, reported no significant difference in students' report of use of alcohol, binge drinking, tobacco, marijuana, or inhalants (Valente et al., 2022). The authors suggested reconsideration of the program before further implementation. On the other hand, a translation of the same program into Spanish has been widely implemented elsewhere in Latin America; Marsiglia et al. (2025) report, in a study with random assignment of schools, significant favorable effects upon cigarette use, marijuana/hard drug use, drug use personal norms, and drug offers from peers. In this version, the curriculum was delivered by classroom teachers trained in a 2-day workshop.

Another widely researched preventive program is Life Skills Training, referred to as a cognitive-behavioral approach, authored and tested by Gilbert Botvin and colleagues. This curriculum teaches general mental health skills as well as domain-specific skills regarding substance use. The results are reported as positive. For example, Botvin et al. (1990) reported on an intervention delivered, not by police, but by regular classroom teachers who had been supplied with the curriculum and trained in a 1-day workshop with some follow-up. The intervention, relative to randomized controls, had significant effects on cigarette smoking, marijuana use, and immoderate alcohol use. A follow-up study (Griffin et al., 2023) of the same participants 13 years later demonstrated significant differences between intervention and control participants with regard to marijuana use, marijuana intoxication, non-medical pill use, and "overall illicit drug use." The difference in drug use among young adults who had received training versus those who had not was on the order of 3 to 6%, which is not a huge effect; however, the fact that significant differences could still be found 13 years after a junior high school intervention is impressive.

"Unplugged" is another program widely implemented and researched in Europe (European Union Drugs Agency, 2025). It is described as "focusing on critical thinking, decision making, problem solving, creative thinking, effective communication, interpersonal relationship skills, self-awareness, empathy, coping with emotions and stress, normative beliefs, and a knowledge about the harmful health effects of drugs." (The phrase "normative beliefs" refers to combating the belief that "everybody" else uses drugs, including alcohol and tobacco, but that substantial numbers avoid them.) The curriculum is delivered by classroom teachers who have been trained for 2.5 days. The students, usually about 11 to 14 years old, experience 12 1-h sessions. Its effects have been assessed in several trials, including a randomized study involving 7079 students in seven countries; significantly positive effects were found at the 15-month follow-up on drunkenness, alcohol-related problems, and cannabis use (Vigna-Taglianti et al., 2014).

We have previously mentioned the Good Behavior Game, which targeted aggressive and disruptive behavior in first and second graders. A total of 1196 children were in the original study (Kellam et al., 2014). The investigators managed to keep up with the participants well enough to follow up with 76% of them when they had reached age 19–21, and conducted a 90-min phone interview. Nineteen percent of males who received the intervention had a lifetime rate of drug abuse and dependence disorder, as contrasted with 38% of the control males. For males who were aggressive and disruptive up to their high school years, 66% of the control group members had drug abuse or dependence at some time, as contrasted with 28% of the Good Behavior Game group (Kellam et al., 2014). There was no specific drug-related content for this intervention; rather, the idea is that aggressive, disruptive behavior is an antecedent for many future problems, including those of substance abuse.

Cochrane reviews of school programs to prevent alcohol abuse (Foxcroft et al., 2011) or other substance abuse (Faggiano et al., 2014) have reported on 51 and 54 studies, respectively, selected from a much larger number. The results are quite inconsistent and difficult to summarize. For example, in the Faggiano review, looking at marijuana use more than 12 months after intervention, of seven studies assessing this, two were significant favoring the intervention; three were non-significant; one was significant favoring the control group; and one showed a "trend" favoring the control group.

So, if one were asked to testify under oath, and a frowning interrogator were to ask, "Is psychoeducation effective for reducing substance use problems? That's a yes or no question; just answer yes or no." We would have to explain that this question cannot be answered yes or no. The word *psychoeducation* is so heterogeneous that it applies to widely varying programs administered with widely varying fidelity and doses, and the recipients and their environments vary widely also. However, it is remarkable and promising that some interventions of relatively few hours, even for the lengthiest of them, have been documented to have positive effects measurable years later. It is also noteworthy that three of the apparently most successful interventions, i.e., Life Skills Training, Unplugged, and the Good Behavior Game, have not restricted themselves to saying no to drugs, but appear to have exerted positive effects mediated by more general social and emotional competence, i.e., by helping kids to be mentally healthier overall.

8.7 Psychoeducation for Social Relationships

What do people do to have happy relationships? There are many answers. They have enjoyable social conversations. They start and finish conversations appropriately, respond on topic to the other, engage in reasonable turn-taking and giving a turn to the other, and use appropriate eye contact. They tell about their own experience and listen empathically and with interest to the other's experience. The music of their tones of voice and vocal inflections communicates approval and enthusiasm. They are kind and helpful. They are able to state their own wishes and needs, using assertion rather than silent resentment or aggressive language. When there are joint decisions or conflicts, they rationally listen to each other's point of view, generate options, think about the pros and cons of the options, and try to pick an option or set of them that takes into account the wishes and needs of each. They minimize commands, criticisms, contradictions, and threats, and maximize reflections, self-disclosures, facilitations (uh huh, yes, I see, OK,...) and positive feedback. They have a high ratio of approving communications to disapproving ones. They avoid raising voices in anger, and they particularly avoid physical violence. They pay attention to the things they can do to make the other person feel valued (channels for value messages) and they try to do those things. They have a repertoire of mutually gratifying activities, i.e., things to do together that both enjoy. They avoid being overly controlling with the other person. They avoid maladaptive jealousy and possessiveness. They are loyal to one another rather than dropping the other when other people or activities command their attention. All of these skills have been components of at least some psychoeducational programs.

A teachable behavior pattern, related to the skills of kindness and approval and positive conversation and mutually gratifying activities, mentioned above, has been emphasized in the research of John Gottman and Julie Schwartz Gottman: the response of someone to the other person's bids for connection. That is, people communicate wishes for interaction and responsiveness by words, touches, facial expressions and gestures, and other behaviors; the person who receives this bid can turn toward it, i.e., reinforce it; turn away from it, i.e., avoid responding to it; or turn against it, i.e., respond with irritation and disapproval. These responses to the other's bids predicted the long-term outcome of the relationship: happy couples "turned toward" 86% of the time whereas those destined for divorce did so only 33% of the time (Gottman, 1994a, 1994b). A 2-day workshop on relationship skills for couples, based on this and other skills, was followed by increased marital satisfaction, better friendship quality, and less destructive conflict at 1-year follow-up. For most measures, this was true no matter whether there was emphasis on friendship enhancement or conflict management in the intervention, although the group where psychoeducation included both seemed to benefit from the broader curriculum (Babcock et al., 2013). Regarding our concern with scalability: another group's intervention consisted solely of bibliotherapy regarding the same content, i.e., provision of the book, *The Seven Principles for Making Marriage Work* (Gottman & Silver, 1999), without the investigators even asking whether the participants read the book. This group also did quite well on several measures, and improvement was not statistically different from the other groups.

The Family Check-Up is an example of an intervention of several components. The intervention is based in middle schools; there are parts offered universally and parts offered to solve target problems. The intervention with both parents and adolescents aims at reducing coercive interactions, promoting positive behavior support, monitoring of adolescent behavior, limit setting, and family problem-solving. Parent work is drawn from the *Everyday Parenting* curriculum (Dishion et al., 2011). Components are delivered in proportion to the assessed need for them in the family in question. The average intervention family in a trial of this received about 6 h of intervention time. This intervention was found to favorably affect several adolescent outcomes, including high-risk sexual behavior, substance use, antisocial behavior, and depression (Fosco et al., 2016).

A review and meta-analysis of family-based prevention programs for adolescent substance abuse (Van Ryzin, 2016) identified, as a component contributing to efficacy, interactions with youth that are meant to improve family relations, such as an exercise in which adolescents are asked to think about issues and conflicts from their parents' perspective.

For many people with a diagnosis of autism spectrum disorder, social skills problems are the major reasons for impairment. One highly researched program for social skills training with autistic folks is called PEERS: Program for the Education and Enrichment of Relational Skills (Laugeson & Frankel, 2010). Chien et al. (2023) cite ten clinical trials of PEERS training, and in addition report on a trial of a translation of this curriculum into Mandarin, tested in Taiwan. The intervention produced positive effects on various measures of social skill, as well as a global measure of autism severity.

8.8 Psychoeducation for Schizophrenia and Other Severe and Psychotic Disorders

One might think that schizophrenia is a disorder where the medical model reigns supreme, and psychoeducation is irrelevant. Toward the end of his life, Aaron Beck turned his attention to using cognitive behavior therapy with schizophrenic patients, with quite positive results: Rector and Beck (2012) reported that cognitive behavior therapy produced large clinical effects on both positive and negative symptoms of schizophrenia. A Cochrane review (Xia et al., 2011) reported that psychoeducation (in the narrower sense than we have used it, i.e., teaching patients about their illness and its treatment) reduced hospital readmissions and relapses, and improved global functioning. Psychoeducation for family members, including teaching about lowering "expressed emotion" (the unfortunately named label for bossiness and hostile criticism), indeed resulted in behavior in caregivers that would appear to improve emotional climate, and improved treatment adherence in patients (Budiono et al., 2021).

An interesting niche of work with schizophrenic individuals concerns auditory hallucinations. The major problem with auditory hallucinations for many or most patients is not the fact that they are experienced as heard rather than just thought, but the content of what the voices say, which is often very hostile and critical and gives directives to do very unwise things. What if people can train their voices to be kinder and wiser—might that perhaps even do more good than trying to get rid of them? A number of interventions have used this strategy with positive result (Craig et al., 2018; Mayhew & Gilbert, 2008; Chadwick & Birchwood, 1994). The Mayhew and Gilbert (2008) study reported, for example, that "All participants' auditory hallucinations became less malevolent, less persecuting and more reassuring." Although these studies so far have been in a treatment context rather than a preventive psychoeducation context, it is not too big a leap to presume that training in self-nurturing, self-reinforcing, and rational self-talk would improve the prognosis of those disposed to become schizophrenic.

Regarding bipolar disorder, Social Rhythm Therapy, as developed by Ellen Frank and often combined with Interpersonal therapy, has produced positive effects in two controlled trials reviewed by Frank et al. (2007). This therapy is based on the idea that regular circadian rhythms are important to maintain, especially in people with bipolar disorder. Haynes et al. (2016) reviewed other studies, including one in which improvement in social rhythm stability was correlated with improvement in PTSD symptoms. These interventions have been carried out in treatment settings and not preventive settings, but the educational nature of the intervention and the high prevalence of circadian rhythm problems in adolescents suggest that such training would be a useful part of preventive psychoeducation.

8.9 SEL (Social and Emotional Learning in Schools)

The notion of starting from an early age and teaching children, in schools, how to be mentally healthy, is not new. Plato wrote about the necessity of early training of children, positive choices for stories they were exposed to, and provision of character-enhancing experiences in games. Religions of all varieties have taken on the task of teaching virtuous behavior to children and youth. One of the early applications of social science to preventive mental health was the Interpersonal Cognitive Problem Solving program (now known as I Can Problem Solve) (Shure & Spivack, 1979, 1980, 1982). This program emphasizes generation of options for choices and teaches young children the vocabulary and concepts helpful in good decision-making. How to think, rather than what to think, has been a watchword in this program.

I Can Problem Solve is one of 99 different programs listed by CASEL, the Collaborative for Academic, Social, and Emotional Learning (2026). References for the effectiveness evaluations of each of these programs are listed.

There has been remarkable growth in the adoption of SEL curricula since about 2010. As of the 2023–2024 school year, CASEL reported that 83% of school principals reported that their schools used an SEL curriculum. This is despite legislative proposals in nine states opposing such curricula.

What has been taught? A number of programs have organized around, or at least overlapped with, five clusters of competences identified by CASEL: self-awareness, self-management, social awareness, relationship skills, and responsible decision-making (Greenberg, 2023).

How effective has such training been? Greenberg (2023) reviewed 12 meta-analyses, and tabulated effect sizes for different outcomes. As an example, a meta-analysis by Durlak et al. (2022) reported the following effect sizes, in standardized mean difference units, from 213 studies of K-12 grade interventions: SEL skills, 0.57; positive social behaviors, 0.24; reduced conduct problems, 0.22; reduced emotional distress, 0.24; and academic success, 0.27. Another meta-analysis (Cipriano et al., 2023) of 424 studies from 53 countries, with about 575,000 students, reported effect sizes in the 0.2 region for SEL skills, attitudes and beliefs, prosocial behaviors, and externalizing behaviors. The highest effect size in this study, about 0.3, was for school climate and safety. Mahoney et al. (2018) reviewed research on SEL programs, including four meta-analyses. Modest but significant results are reported both at post-intervention and at follow-up for positive social behaviors, conduct problems, emotional distress, and academic performance.

A small statistical digression is in order in digesting the results of meta-analyses. Greenberg (2023) use a revised definition of effect size cutoffs based on a review of 747 clinical trials in education by Kraft (2019). Kraft argued that effect sizes of 0.05 to 0.20 should be called medium, and those over 0.20 should be called large, because of the distribution of effect sizes found in education; also, because smaller effect sizes are of greater importance when they result from interventions scaled over large numbers of recipients. The cutoffs differ greatly from those proposed by Jacob Cohen (1988) of 0.2, 0.5, and 0.8 for small, medium, and large, respectively, for standard deviation differences in means. Kraft's revision is, of course, debatable. The fact remains that with normal distributions in experimental and control groups, the probability that a random experimental subject will fare better than a random control subject increases from 50% (for a zero effect size) to 51.4% for a 0.05 effect, to 55.6% for a 0.20 effect. The probability reaches 76% at a 1.0 effect size. (These are from calculations explained in elementary statistics courses.) When many people read that children in the experimental group did better on a certain outcome, they imagine that almost all of them did better; this becomes true only with very large effect sizes. Improving the chances of superiority from 50% to a little over 55.6% arguably is not compatible with most people's image of a large effect. Nonetheless, even if we balk at redefining the words describing effect sizes, we should be aware that small effect sizes are very much worth attaining in interventions that are quite scalable and are free of side effects; also we should not expect large effect sizes from universal interventions on measures of psychopathology, since effect sizes will be diluted by many students who would not meet the threshold of psychopathology with or without the intervention.

Given the great importance of kindness as a habit that contributes not only to the mental health of the doer of kind acts, but also to the recipients, it is important that SEL programs are having success in teaching kindness, a.k.a. prosocial behavior. Schonert-Reichl et al. (2015) describe a curriculum used with fourth and fifth graders which the authors describe as mindfulness-based, but also emphasized seeing things from others' perspectives, feeling gratitude, and carrying out kind acts. In a randomized study, students who received the intervention reported improvement relative to controls with respect to various self-reported aspects of mental health, peer ratings of prosocial behavior and aggression, and of stress physiology as measured by salivary cortisol.

We include, in the discussion of SEL, efforts to teach school children to tutor other children—of same-age peers, or younger children in "cross-age tutoring." Shi & Cheung's, 2024 meta-analysis reported that cross-age tutoring had an average effect size of 0.33 for tutees, and 0.39 for tutors, with respect to academic outcomes. This study reported the unsurprising, but important, observation that programs with larger doses of intervention tended to have larger effect sizes. With respect to social and psychological outcomes, a meta-analysis by Burton et al. (2021) reported that effect sizes of cross-age tutoring for these outcomes were not significantly different from those for academic outcomes; the overall effect size averaged across all outcomes in this study was 0.45. This meta-analysis reported that among the moderating variables appearing to affect outcomes were the amount of pre-match training of tutors, the frequency of meetings, and the level of adult oversight. The empirical data appear to support the notion that "The more you put into it, the more you get out of it."

One of the most ambitious, thorough, innovative, and ground-breaking school interventions was described by Gerald Newmark, 50 years before the time of this writing (1976). The intervention aimed to transform the entire school culture. At the heart was cross-age tutoring; teachers of younger and older classrooms were paired, and the older children tutored the younger ones. At first, the content was very circumscribed and scripted; as time went by, more and more of the school curriculum was handled via tutoring. The democratic process was adopted to give students and all staff, together, experience in shared planning and decision-making. Parents who could be available were enlisted in the cause of tutoring and helping with the various tasks of education. And in groups, students, teachers, and administrators gave open feedback to one another about what was going on in the school. The outcome reporting was all anecdotal rather than statistical, but it makes a convincing case, and represents a remarkable feat of cooperation by many people to get on board with new ways of doing things.

8.10 Efforts toward Mental Health in the Workplace

Since most adults spend a high fraction of their waking hours in workplaces, it stands to reason that the quality of the work environment is a very important determinant of health, including mental health. Tinson (2020) reported that UK employees with aspects of low quality work, categorized as jobs low in autonomy, satisfaction, well-being, pay, and security, reported worse health status. Only 27% of workers surveyed reported none of these five problematic conditions. Low job well-being was defined as whether the job inspired "tension, unease, worry, depression, gloom, or misery."

Numerous interventions have been used to promote workplace mental health. Wu et al. (2021) reviewed findings on best practices; these were used to create an award (the Mattingly Award, given by a partnership of the Johns Hopkins School of Public Health and the Luv u Foundation) meant to incentivize positive workplace practices. Some of these practices are a culture that values mental health; attempts to reduce stress in the workplace; mental health training for workers, including stress management; programs to prevent bullying, harassment, and incivility; opportunities to mentally recharge (break rooms, time off); opportunities for social connection; training of leadership in supportive supervision and reasonable and clear performance expectations; and measurement of employee well-being outcomes. Hesketh et al. (2021) reviewed many studies and several meta-analyses, of workplace interventions; many positive effects, along with several insignificant effects, are reported; the authors remark that effect sizes are often small. Demou et al. (2024) reviewed 20 studies of group-level (as contrasted with individual-level) workplace interventions. Thirteen of these measured mental health outcomes; of these, nine reported positive and significant effects, and four reported no significant difference between experimental and control groups. A 2025 review by Abraham et al. of workplace interventions for university staff noted that the ordinary workload itself interfered with devoting more time during work hours to mental health intervention, and moving interventions to time outside the ordinary work hours did not satisfactorily solve this problem.

A summary figure about the average effect size of workplace interventions for mental health would be meaningless or misleading, because there is such great heterogeneity in workplaces, in intervention components, in the personalities of those facilitating and receiving interventions, and in the overall economic conditions of the industry involved. Nonetheless, the empirical work on workplace mental health, combined with many hours spent by authors of this book listening to psychotherapy clients describing mental health consequences of poor emotional climates in the workplace (especially punitive, rather than educative, behaviors of bosses) make the point convincingly that the workplace as an arena for mental health promotion should not be neglected.

8.11 Recovery International, 12 Step Groups, and Other Peer-Led Self-Help

The most famous mutual aid group is surely Alcoholics Anonymous (AA). AA was formed in the USA in the 1930s with origins in Christian revivals. It is "psychoeducational" in that its goal is for members to learn new patterns of healthy living and sobriety. There are some written texts, of which the two most prominent are *Alcoholics Anonymous*, otherwise known as the *Big Book* (Alcoholics Anonymous World Services, 2001), and *Twelve Steps and Twelve Traditions* (Alcoholics Anonymous World Services, 1981). (The full texts of these are available at AA.org.) The 12 steps taught by AA are strongly based on transformation through spirituality. The 12 steps involve (1) admitting powerlessness over alcohol; (2) concluding that a higher power could restore mental health; (3) turning over our lives to the higher power; (4) making a fearless moral inventory of ourselves; (5) admitting to God, ourselves, and someone else our wrongdoings; (6) becoming ready to have God improve us; (7) asking Him to remove our shortcomings; (8) listing people we've harmed, so as to consider restitution; (9) following through with restitution when reasonable; (10) continuing to take inventory and admit our mistakes; (11) praying to learn God's will and to carry it out; and (12) helping other alcoholics and practicing these principles in general conduct of life. Despite the strong religious content of the 12 steps, AA does not require membership or allegiance to any religious organization; membership is open to all and meetings and sponsorship are provided without cost. The AA traditions discourage property acquisition by the organization and contributions from non-members. The activities are organized around group meetings; each group is able to determine the content. Perhaps the most central activity is first-person accounts by members of their experiences, and mutual support by group members. Sponsorship, or mentorship, of newer members by members who have maintained sobriety, can involve interactions that go on outside meetings. Alcoholics Anonymous has spawned other 12 step groups for other problems: narcotics anonymous, overeaters anonymous, gamblers, debtors, sex and love addicts … at least 28 groups (Leurent et al., 2024).

Alcoholics Anonymous certainly meets the criterion of scalability: around 2 million people are estimated to be members, mostly in the USA and Canada, but also in several other countries. And it is delivered at zero cost to either taxpayers or health insurance companies—it has been called a "free lunch" for public health. A 2020 Cochrane review (Kelly et al., 2020) reported both on the results of a manualized version of AA, suitable for randomized clinical trials, and on the usual non-manualized version. Although the degree of detail in this review is hard to summarize succinctly, suffice it to say that AA compared favorably with other interventions such as cognitive behavior therapy and motivational enhancement therapy. For the manualized interventions, about 42% of AA participants were completely abstinent at 1-year follow-up, as contrasted to about 35% of participants in other clinical interventions.

Many people find the admission of powerlessness over alcohol and seeing the source of deliverance from addiction in a higher power to be antithetical to their philosophies. Accordingly, secular mutual aid groups for help with alcohol have grown up; one of the most prominent is Smart Recovery. Smart Recovery emphasizes that power resides within human beings to break addictions, with the help of mutual support and any findings that science has to offer. Kelly et al. (2023) describe an ongoing study in which participants are not randomized, but select for themselves whether to participate in Smart Recovery, Alcoholics Anonymous, both, or neither. At 6 months, on most measures, Smart Recovery appeared to perform at least as well as AA. The percent totally abstinent at 6 months was about 14% with Smart Recovery and about 11% with AA (Kelly et al., 2026). These results remind us of two truisms: outcome studies are highly dependent upon the sample entering the study, and addiction to alcohol is not easy to solve.

There are mutual aid groups for the alleviation of psychopathology other than addiction. One of the earliest and longest-lasting is currently called Recovery International, previously called Recovery Inc., which began in 1937. This organization is peer-led, secular, and offered at no cost. Regarding education, the members of this organization study and read aloud to each other in meetings a manual by Abraham Low, *Mental Health Through Will-Training* (Low, 1950). Low's teachings overlap greatly with what later came to be called cognitive behavior therapy. In meetings, members speak of upsetting events, identify the thoughts or attitudes that contributed to the upset, and use Dr. Low's ideas, including a set of maxims, in thought revision. Recovery International uses the word "endorse" to refer to people's complimenting, congratulating, or reinforcing themselves or others for positive handlings of situations. The word "will" was apparently chosen to emphasize that conscious, deliberate decision-making could prevail in reducing symptoms, as contrasted with the primacy of the unconscious. Galanter (1988) reported on an observational study of this organization, including that about half of the members were hospitalized psychiatrically before joining, whereas under a tenth were hospitalized after starting to participate; the need for psychiatric treatment in general appeared to diminish as a function of the time members had participated. Recovery International, despite being based on sound principles, and being another "free lunch" for public health, has not generated as much research activity or total participation as some of the 12 step groups have.

8.12 A Word about Religion

Volumes have been written about religion and its effects. Because religious practices are so heterogeneous, it's not meaningful to pose the question, "What are the mental health effects of religion?" But there have even been randomized controlled trials of specific religious practices, done for a specified length of time (e.g., Plante et al., 2025).

We are not ambitious enough (and there is not space enough) to tackle this subject. Suffice it to make some brief observations. First, for centuries, it has been the bailiwick of at least a portion of religious practice to attempt to elicit compassion and ethical behavior, a sense of meaning and purpose, and joyful feelings including gratitude, which are important parts of mental health and targets of psychoeducation. Second, participation in organized religion has declined significantly in the USA in recent decades (Smith, 2025); the decline in Europe is probably even greater (Molteni & Biolcati, 2023). Thus, the hypothesis comes to mind (and we'll not attempt to prove or disprove it) that the decline in religion leaves a void in the total number of hours society is devoting to the abovementioned goals, which have not been filled by a compensatory rise in secular programs. Third, an almost universal problem of psychoeducational programs is that "time on task" is too small to make a big difference. Religious institutions allocate time in a dramatically different way, expecting, demanding, or at least making available, some time each week (if not daily) over the course of a lifetime. Given forgetting curves for any sort of educational experience, it could be that for psychoeducation to bring forth maximal fruits, a similar never-ending model may be more in keeping with the nature of human beings. As an example, it's exciting to envision a culture in which most adults routinely would spend half an hour with a child each day in psychoeducation, for the benefit of the adult as well as the child. (It's another thing entirely to actually cause such a culture to come about!)

8.13 The Mass Media: Psychoeducation for Better or for Worse

Education, broadly defined, is influence toward learning, using any of the methods of influence enumerated in a previous chapter—modeling, reinforcement (including vicarious reinforcement), practice (including fantasy practice), objective-formation (including the sales pitches of attractive people), and others. Viewed in this way, it is almost impossible for a human being to encounter another without influencing or educating at least a little, whether the encounter is in real life or via print or electronic communications. For example, every behavior we witness is a model; every thing that anyone does is either pleasant, unpleasant, or neutral, and thus provides reinforcement, non-reinforcement, or punishment. As countless research studies have shown, what comes to us via the media influences us.

The sheer quantity of influence provided through mass media dwarfs the amount of time spent in most "interventions" that have been meticulously designed, tried, analyzed, and meta-analyzed. For adolescents in the USA, estimates as large as 6 to 9 h a day have been reported for total screen use (Santos et al., 2023). Since it was first published in 1980, David Burns's mass market explication of cognitive behavior therapy, in various editions, has sold over 4 million copies—by any criteria for books, a best-seller (Burns, 2026). By contrast, various versions of Call of Duty, a first-person shooter game, have sold about 500 million copies since the first version in 2003 until 2024 (Guinness World Records, 2024). Similar numbers apply to Grand Theft Auto, whose first-person anti-heroes in addition to shooting can do lots of other antisocial activities, including rape, stabbing, and running people over with vehicles. The global annual revenue from first-person shooter games was estimated at about 29 billion US dollars in 2023 (Zion Market Research, 2026) and 34 billion as of 2026 (Business Research Insights, 2026). An Internet site posts Call of Duty players' lifetime numbers of "kills" (COD Stats Tracker, 2026). Of 300 players whose statistics are posted, each of them individually had accumulated over 200,000 kills, and one player reportedly had accumulated over 2 billion kills. (The psychometric reliability and validity of these "kill" figures are not reported!)

A meta-analysis by Anderson et al. (2010) found significant effects (in the direction expected by modeling and fantasy rehearsal principles) of video game violence upon aggressive behavior, cognition, and emotion; empathy versus desensitization to others' distress; and on prosocial behavior. Effect sizes were in the small region, i.e., around 0.2 correlation coefficient units (0.1 = small effect, 0.3 = moderate). The authors point out that in a multidetermined phenomenon such as aggression, no one factor is expected to account for a large fraction of the variance; the effect size for video game violence is in about the same ball park as substance abuse, poverty, and abusive parents (Anderson et al., 2010, p. 170).

The hypothesis that media violence increases real-life aggressive and mean behavior has been the subject of hundreds of research studies, reviewed by Anderson et al. (2016), summarized as follows: "After decades of research a clear finding emerges: violent media exposure is a causal risk factor for increases in aggression." As an example of the research still accumulating, Huesmann et al. (2021) found, in a longitudinal study of children, that more violent video game experience predicted, 10 years later, more gun use or threats to use weapons, and more beliefs in favor of gun use.

The connection between violent video games and subsequent aggression has been debated, with the "no effect" position argued primarily by Ferguson and colleagues (e.g., Elson & Ferguson, 2014). One of the issues debated is whether "nonserious" aggression, i.e., aggressive attitudes and talk, should be excluded from analyses. A meta-analysis by Prescott et al. (2018) addressed some of the objections presented by Ferguson, but still found a significant relation between time 1 violent video game playing and time 2 overt physical aggression.

Immersing oneself in this debate offers a chance to learn much about research design, meta-analysis, and effect sizes. But another way of thinking about media violence (as well as abusive talk and other forms of exploitation and cruelty in media) is to appreciate the power of both imitation learning (or modeling) and fantasy rehearsal as basic mechanisms for why people do what they do. Modeling and imitation learning were studied extensively by Albert Bandura, not just by his famous Bobo doll experiment (Bandura et al., 1961). These influences on learning are reckoned with in almost all theories of learning (Kymissis & Poulson, 1990). A 2020 meta-analysis of 88 studies with over 25,000 participants (Jung et al., 2020) reported an effect size of 0.45 for the effectiveness of presenting prosocial models in promoting prosocial behavior in observers. Fantasy rehearsal, a.k.a. imaginal exposure, has been a mainstay in the treatment of phobias and anxiety disorders at least since the seminal work of Joseph Wolpe (1969). A meta-analysis of virtual reality exposures for anxiety disorders reported a large effect size ($g = 0.90$) when compared with waitlist, and a Hedge's g of 0.78 when compared with psychological placebo, with insignificant differences between virtual and real-life exposure methods (Carl et al., 2019). Fantasy rehearsal has been reported to have effects in the expected direction (i.e., the same as real-life practice) for learning surgical skills (Anton et al., 2017), music performance (Bernardi et al., 2013), and dance performance (Abraham et al., 2016). In 1972, Richard Suinn reported that ski racers who rehearsed the ski run in fantasy did better upon subsequent timing than controls. By the 1988 Olympics, 93% of Olympic athletes used some form of fantasy rehearsal to maximize performance (Ungerleider & Golding, 1991). A 2025 meta-analysis of 86 studies with over 3500 athletes (Liu et al., 2025) found an overall effect size of 0.5 for "imagery practice" on athletic performance. The point of all this is that if modeling and fantasy rehearsal influence behaviors as widely varied as kicking dolls, tennis playing, getting over fears of flying, performing surgery, playing the violin, and dancing, it strains credulity to think that models and rehearsals of aggressive and cruel behavior somehow are immune to being affected.

As if the negative influence of video games (on top of that of violent television and movies) were not enough, the experience of childhood and adolescence has been dramatically altered by the advent of smartphones and social media. Jonathan Haidt (2024) is a widely known proponent of the idea that childhood centering around smartphones since about 2010 has brought on a surge in adolescent and young adult mental health problems. He lists four foundational harms: social deprivation, resulting from the diversion of attention from face to face interactions with friends to online interactions with relatively anonymous people; sleep deprivation, resulting from how hard it is to resist temptations coming via phone after bedtime; attention fragmentation, resulting from how easy it is to flip to something new on the phone; and addiction, resulting from the fact that very smart people have worked intensely to make phone attractions that are difficult to resist, and from the fact that the phone is always available as a source of gratification. We can propose another source of harm: it appears to be easier for people to be cruel to one another when they are not face to face. Both those practicing cruelty and those receiving it are having mental health harmed.

This chapter has reviewed a number of very promising psychoeducational interventions. But the number of hours that these interventions are experienced is dwarfed by the number of hours young people are spending with videogames, movies, TV, and social media. Society must confront the fact that the mass media are "psychoeducational interventions" themselves, for better or for worse. They provide models, reinforcement contingencies, opportunities for practice, and sometimes explicit instruction. They induce motivation for change in a certain direction; they provide stimuli which bring out certain behaviors; they make relationships available—in short, they can provide each of the ten OH RAM PRISM influence methods we discussed earlier. Users cannot avoid learning from these influences.

8.14 Telephone Tutoring in Reading and Psychological Skills

We may close this chapter on an optimistic note, noting that the sheer volume of published research on psychoeducation is almost overwhelming. Indeed, stopping citing research is more based on "We have to stop somewhere" than "We've covered all the relevant research." Outcomes are very predominantly positive despite relatively lower times on task than most other educational enterprises.

In addition, to cite some "lived experience" conducting psychoeducation: one of us (Strayhorn, 2016) has been developing a psychoeducational intervention for about three decades. Non-professionals, mainly college students, but also some high school students and some older adults, are trained to deliver psychoeducation to children (and occasionally adolescents) in half-hour phone sessions occurring five or six times a week, for at least a year and sometimes as many as 3 or 4 years. (The "time on task" issue is taken seriously.) The program started out as a reading tutoring program; students who had progressed at 0.44 grade equivalents per year prior to tutoring advanced to an average of 2.0 grade equivalents per year during tutoring (Strayhorn, 2005). Since 2001, over 20 manuals have been added to the armamentarium for the program, on skills such as self-discipline, friendship-building, anxiety reduction, conflict resolution and anger control, why and how to do psychological skills exercises, and so forth. (These are currently available in full text at josephstrayhornmd.com.) As the students practice reading, they simultaneously read models and instructions on psychological skills. Most of the manuals have been written in a "programmed" format tailored for tutoring: there are numbered sections of about 200 words, followed by an A or B comprehension probe. In "alternate reading," the tutor and student take turns reading the sections aloud to one another; the student answers the comprehension probe; the tutor gets to reinforce the student for the correct answer at least 80% of the time. (If the student performs below this level, they should usually move "down the hierarchy" to simpler reading material.) This format has proved to increase student engagement greatly compared to straight exposition. In alternate reading, the student can work on psychological skills while at the same time practicing the most important academic skill, reading comprehension. After a few minutes in alternate reading, the tutor and student spend some time doing psychological skills exercises as outlined in the previous chapter. And part of the session is devoted to social conversation, given the importance of this skill in relationships and life. So far, only anecdotal evidence for effectiveness in psychological growth has accumulated, but many anecdotes are of positive changes to the life trajectory. A few students who were on the verge of being expelled from schools because of aggression gradually eliminated problematic aggression. (Lots of fantasy rehearsals of hypothetical provocations were presumably major contributors to these changes.) Some students with disabling compulsive symptoms became nearly compulsion-free off medication. (Daily readings of fantasy rehearsals of exposure and ritual prevention were key.) Children who hated school have changed their attitudes once they became much more competent at reading. Children with social anxiety and social skills problems have made friends (both structured and unstructured practice in social conversation appeared to contribute). Children with work aversions have learned to enjoy working, probably because of experiences doing work that was adjusted to be neither too hard nor too easy, and with feedback on results over time. Students with panic attacks have become panic-free, having read about anti-hyperventilation exercises, among other strategies, and practiced them with their tutors. Students with dangerous behaviors that appeared to be motivated by a wish to be noticed have ceased those behaviors upon having one-to-one undivided attention for a half hour daily. And hopefully, almost all of them have come to value acts of kindness and productivity at least a little more than before, and to feel joyous about each of their accomplishments in these realms. Quantitative outcome study of this program has been planned, and research support has been applied for. Some anecdotal data also suggests that the program may have a positive effect on tutors—the principles are applicable to people of all ages, and the tutor and student learn together. In addition, the interpersonal skills emphasized for tutors overlap greatly with those taught for positive parenting, couple relationships, friendships, and work supervision, including skills of creating a positive emotional climate. The telephone tutoring bypasses many logistic and political issues that would need to be surmounted for, say, widespread tutoring of elementary school children by high schoolers using the same methods and materials during school days or after school programs. But the methods and materials are available either for use by schools or for telephone tutoring on a larger scale, and researchers and practitioners are invited to explore such methods further and build upon what has been done so far.

References

Abraham, A., Dunsky, A., & Dickstein, R. (2016). Motor imagery practice for enhancing elevé performance among professional dancers: A pilot study. *Medical Problems of Performing Artists, 31*, 132–139.

Abraham, J., Smith, L., O'Donnell, C., & Patel, R. (2025). Workplace mental health interventions for university staff: A systematic review of effectiveness and implementation challenges. *Journal of Occupational Health Psychology, 30*(2), 145–162.

Ackerson, J., Scogin, F., McKendree-Smith, N., & Lyman, R. D. (1998). Cognitive bibliotherapy for mild and moderate adolescent depressive symptomatology. *Journal of Consulting and Clinical Psychology, 66*(4), 685–690. https://doi.org/10.1037/0022-006X.66.4.685

Alcoholics Anonymous World Services. (1981). Twelve steps and twelve traditions.

Alcoholics Anonymous World Services. (2001). *Alcoholics Anonymous* (4th ed.).

American Academy of Sleep Medicine. (2023). *Sleep prioritization survey: Sleep aid use*. https://www.aasm.org/wp-content/uploads/2023/06/sleep-prioritization-survey-2023-sleep-aids.pdf

Anderson, C. A., Shibuya, A., Ihori, N., Swing, E. L., Bushman, B. J., Sakamoto, A., Rothstein, H. R., & Saleem, M. (2010). Violent video game effects on aggression, empathy, and prosocial behavior in eastern and western countries: A meta-analytic review. *Psychological Bulletin, 136*(2), 151–173. https://doi.org/10.1037/a0018251

Anderson, C. A., Groves, C. L., & Prot, S. (2016). Violent media effects: Current theory and evidence. An update. In C. L. Groves, S. Prot, & C. A. Anderson (Eds.), *Violent media effects: Theory and evidence. In H. S. Friedman (Ed) Encyclopedia of Mental Health (Second Edition)* (pp. 362–369). Academic Press. https://doi.org/10.1016/B978-0-12-397045-9.00257-3. Available at https://craiganderson.org/wp-content/uploads/caa/abstracts/2020-2024/22AGP.pdf

Anderson, L., Lewis, G., Araya, R., Elgie, R., Harrison, G., Proudfoot, J., Schmidt, U., Sharp, D., Weightman, A., & Williams, C. (2005). Self-help books for depression: How can practitioners and patients make the right choice? *The British Journal of General Practice, 55*(514), 387–392.

Anton, N. E., Bean, E. A., Hammonds, S. C., & Stefanidis, D. (2017). Application of mental skills training in surgery: A review of its effectiveness and proposed next steps. *Journal of Laparoendoscopic & Advanced Surgical Techniques, 27*, 459–469.

Babcock, J. C., Gottman, J. M., Ryan, K. D., & Gottman, J. S. (2013). A randomized clinical trial of relationship enhancement and conflict management interventions for couples. *Journal of Family Psychology, 27*(4), 625–635.

Bandura, A., Ross, D., & Ross, S. A. (1961). Transmission of aggression through imitation of aggressive models. *Journal of Abnormal and Social Psychology, 63*, 575–582.

Beck, J. S. (2021). *Cognitive behavior therapy: Basics and beyond* (3rd ed.). Guilford Press.

Bernardi, N. F., De Buglio, M., Trimarchi, P. D., Chielli, A., & Bricolo, E. (2013). Mental practice promotes motor anticipation: Evidence from skilled music performance. *Frontiers in Human Neuroscience, 7*, –451.

Bonin, E. M., Stevens, M., Beecham, J., Byford, S., & Parsonage, M. (2011). Costs and longer-term savings of parenting programmes for the prevention of persistent conduct disorder: A modelling study. *BMC Public Health, 11*, 803. https://doi.org/10.1186/1471-2458-11-803

Botvin, G. J., Baker, E., Dusenbury, L., Tortu, S., & Botvin, E. M. (1990). Preventing adolescent drug abuse through a multimodal cognitive–behavioral approach: Results of a three-year study. *Journal of Consulting and Clinical Psychology, 58*(4), 437–446.

Brown, R. T., D'Emidio-Caston, M., & Pollard, J. A. (1995). Students' perceptions of drug prevention programs: A qualitative and quantitative evaluation of DARE. *Journal of Drug Education, 25*(3), 215–232.

Brunwasser, S. M., Gillham, J. E., & Kim, E. S. (2009). A meta-analytic review of the Penn resiliency program's effect on depressive symptoms. *Journal of Consulting and Clinical Psychology, 77*(6), 1042–1054. https://doi.org/10.1037/a0017671

Budiono, W., Kantono, K., Kristianto, F. C., Avanti, C., & Herawati, F. (2021). Psychoeducation improved illness perception and expressed emotion of family caregivers of patients with schizophrenia. *International Journal of Environmental Research and Public Health, 18*, 7522. https://doi.org/10.3390/ijerph18147522

Burns, D. D. (1980). *Feeling good: The new mood therapy*. HarperCollins.

Burns, D. D. (2026). *Mini description of David's books as well as a comparison table below*. https://feelinggood.com/books.

Burton, E., Anderson, J., Prater, M. A., & Dyches, T. T. (2021). The effects of cross-age tutoring on academic and social outcomes: A systematic review. *Education and Treatment of Children, 44*(2), 123–146.

Business Research Insights. (2026). *FPS game market size, share, growth, and industry analysis, by type*. https://www.businessresearchinsights.com/market-reports/fps-game-market-117646.

Carl, E., Stein, A. T., Levihn-Coon, A., Pogue, J. R., Rothbaum, B., Emmelkamp, P., Asmundson, G. J. G., Carlbring, P., & Powers, M. B. (2019). Virtual reality exposure therapy for anxiety and related disorders: A meta-analysis of randomized controlled trials. *Journal of Anxiety Disorders, 61*, 27–36. https://doi.org/10.1016/j.janxdis.2018.08.003

Chadwick, P., & Birchwood, M. (1994). The omnipotence of voices: A cognitive approach to auditory hallucinations. *The British Journal of Psychiatry, 164*(2), 190–201. https://doi.org/10.1192/bjp.164.2.190

Chapman, A. L., & Gratz, K. L. (2015). *The dialectical behavior therapy skills workbook for anger: Using DBT mindfulness and emotion regulation skills to manage anger*. New Harbinger Publications.

Chien, Y.-L., Gau, S. S.-F., Shang, C.-Y., & Wu, Y.-Y. (2023). A systematic review of the PEERS® social skills training program for autistic adolescents and young adults. *Clinical Child and Family Psychology Review, 26*(3), 543–566.

Cipriano, C., Strambler, M. J., Naples, L. H., Ha, C., Kirk, M., Wood, M., Sehgal, K., Zieher, A. K., Eveleigh, A., McCarthy, M., Funaro, M., Ponnock, A., Chow, J. C., & Durlak, J. (2023). The state of evidence for social and emotional learning: A contemporary meta-analysis of universal school-based SEL interventions. *Child Development, 94*(5). https://doi.org/10.1111/cdev.13962

COD Stats Tracker. (2026). *Kills leaderboards*. http://codstats.net/leaderboards/kills

Cohen, J. (1988). *Statistical power analysis for the behavioral sciences* (2nd ed.). Routledge.

Collaborative for Academic, Social, and Emotional Learning. (2026). *Program guide: Evidence-based social and emotional learning programs*. https://pg.casel.org/review-programs/

Craig, T. K. J., Rus-Calafell, M., Ward, T., et al. (2018). AVATAR therapy for auditory verbal hallucinations in people with psychosis: A single-blind, randomized controlled trial. *The Lancet Psychiatry, 5*(1), 31–40. https://doi.org/10.1016/S2215-0366(17)30427-3

Craske, M. G., Meuret, A. E., Ritz, T., Treanor, M., Dour, H., & Rosenfield, D. (2019). Positive affect treatment for depression and anxiety: A randomized clinical trial for a core feature of anhedonia. *Journal of Consulting and Clinical Psychology, 87*(5), 457–471. https://doi.org/10.1037/ccp0000396

Craske, M. G., Dour, H. J., Treanor, M., & Meuret, A. E. (2022). *Positive affect treatment for depression and anxiety: Therapist guide*. Oxford University Press.

Craske, M. G., Meuret, A. E., Echiverri-Cohen, A., Rosenfield, D., & Ritz, T. (2023). Positive affect treatment targets reward sensitivity: A randomized controlled trial. *Journal of Consulting and Clinical Psychology, 91*(6), 350–366. https://doi.org/10.1037/ccp0000805

Cuijpers, P. (1997). Bibliotherapy in unipolar depression. *Journal of Behavior Therapy and Experimental Psychiatry, 28*, 139–147.

Cuijpers, P. (1998). A psychoeducational approach to the treatment of depression: A meta-analysis of Lewinsohn's "coping with depression" course. *Behavior Therapy, 29*, 521–533.

Davis, J. A. (1965). *Education for positive mental health: A review of existing research and recommendations for future studies*. Aldine.

Day, J. J., & Sanders, M. R. (2018). Do parents benefit from help when completing a self-guided parenting program online? A randomized controlled trial comparing triple p online with and without telephone support. *Behavior Therapy, 49*(6), 1020–1038. https://doi.org/10.1016/j.beth.2018.03.002

de Graaf, I., Speetjens, P., Smit, F., de Wolff, M., & Tavecchio, L. (2008). Effectiveness of the triple P positive parenting program on behavioral problems in children: A meta-analysis. *Behavior Modification, 32*(5), 714–735. https://doi.org/10.1177/0145445508317134

Demou, E., Bhaskar, A., MacLean, A., O'Connor, R., & Macdonald, E. B. (2024). Group-level workplace mental health interventions: A systematic review of effectiveness and implementation factors. *Scandinavian Journal of Work, Environment & Health, 50*(1), 23–38.

den Boer, P. C., Wiersma, D., & Van den Bosch, R. J. (2004). Why is self-help neglected in the treatment of emotional disorders? A meta-analysis. *Psychological Medicine, 34*(6), 959–971. https://doi.org/10.1017/S003329170300179X

DiGiuseppe, R., & Tafrate, R. C. (2003). Anger treatment for adults: A meta-analytic review. *Clinical Psychology: Science and Practice, 10*(1), 70–84. https://doi.org/10.1093/clipsy.10.1.70

Dishion, T. J., Stormshak, E. A., & Kavanagh, K. (2011). *Everyday parenting: A professional's guide to building family management skills*. Research Press.

Durlak, J. A., Mahoney, J. L., & Boyle, A. E. (2022). What we know, and what we need to find out about universal, school-based social and emotional learning programs for children and adolescents. *Psychological Bulletin, 148*(11–12), 765–795. https://doi.org/10.1037/bul0000383

Elson, M., & Ferguson, C. J. (2014). Twenty-five years of research on violence in digital games and aggression: Empirical evidence, perspectives, and a debate gone astray. *European Psychologist, 19*(1), 33–46. https://doi.org/10.1027/1016-9040/a000147

Ennett, S. T., Tobler, N. S., Ringwalt, C. L., & Flewelling, R. L. (1994). How effective is drug abuse resistance education? A meta-analysis of project DARE outcome evaluations. *American Journal of Public Health, 84*(9), 1394–1401.

Espie, C. A., Kyle, S. D., Williams, C., Ong, J. C., Douglas, N. J., Hames, P., & Brown, J. S. (2012). A randomized, placebo-controlled trial of online cognitive behavioral therapy for chronic insomnia disorder delivered via an automated media-rich web application. *Sleep, 35*(6), 769–781. https://doi.org/10.5665/sleep.1872

European Union Drugs Agency. (2025). *Unplugged: Evidence and implementation of a school-based prevention programme in Europe*. Publications Office of the European Union.

Faggiano, F., Minozzi, S., Versino, E., & Buscemi, D. (2014). Universal school-based prevention for illicit drug use. *Cochrane Database of Systematic Reviews, 2014*(1), CD003020. https://doi.org/10.1002/14651858.CD003020.pub3

Fazel, S., Wolf, A., Chang, Z., Larsson, H., Goodwin, G. M., & Lichtenstein, P. (2015). Depression and violence: A Swedish population study. *The Lancet Psychiatry, 2*(3), 224–232. https://doi.org/10.1016/S2215-0366(14)00128-X

Ferracioli-Oda, E., Qawasmi, A., & Bloch, M. H. (2013). Meta-analysis: Melatonin for the treatment of primary sleep disorders. *PloS One, 8*(5), e63773. https://doi.org/10.1371/journal.pone.0063773

Felder, J. N., Epel, E. S., Neuhaus, J., Krystal, A. D., & Prather, A. A. (2020). Efficacy of digital cognitive behavioral therapy for the treatment of insomnia symptoms among pregnant women: A randomized clinical trial. *JAMA Psychiatry, 77*(5), 484–492. https://doi.org/10.1001/jamapsychiatry.2019.4491

Floyd, M., Rohen, N., Shackelford, J. A. M., Hubbard, K. L., Parnell, M. B., Scogin, F., & Coates, A. (2006). Two-year follow-up of bibliotherapy and individual cognitive therapy for depressed older adults. *Behavior Modification, 30*(3), 281–294. https://doi.org/10.1177/0145445503261176

Floyd, M., Scogin, F., McKendree-Smith, N. L., Floyd, D. L., & Rokke, P. D. (2004). Cognitive therapy for depression: A comparison of individual psychotherapy and bibliotherapy for depressed older adults. *Behavior Modification, 28*(2), 297–318. https://doi.org/10.1177/0145445503259284

Forgatch, M. S., & DeGarmo, D. S. (1999). Parenting through change: An effective prevention program for single mothers. *Journal of Consulting and Clinical Psychology, 67*(5), 711–724. https://doi.org/10.1037/0022-006x.67.5.711

Forgatch, M. S., Patterson, G. R., Degarmo, D. S., & Beldavs, Z. G. (2009). Testing the Oregon delinquency model with 9-year follow-up of the Oregon divorce study. *Development and Psychopathology, 21*(2), 637–660. https://doi.org/10.1017/S0954579409000340

Fosco, G. M., Stormshak, E. A., Dishion, T. J., & Winter, C. (2016). Family check-up intervention effects on adolescent arrest trajectories: Variation by developmental subtype. *Journal of Research on Adolescence, 26*(1), 54–68.

Foundations. (2025). *Penn Resilience Programme (UK implementation in primary school).* https://foundations.org.uk/toolkit/guidebook/penn-resilience-programme-uk-implementation-in-primary-school

Foxcroft, D. R., Moreira, M. T., Almeida Santimano, N. M. L., & Smith, L. A. (2011). Social norms information for alcohol misuse in university and college students. *Cochrane Database of Systematic Reviews, 2011*(7), CD006748. https://doi.org/10.1002/14651858.CD006748.pub2

Furlong, M., McGilloway, S., Bywater, T., Hutchings, J., Smith, S. M., & Donnelly, M. (2013). Cochrane review: Behavioural and cognitive-behavioural group-based parenting programmes for early-onset conduct problems in children aged 3 to 12 years (review). *Evidence-Based Child Health: A Cochrane Review Journal, 8*(2), 318–692. https://doi.org/10.1002/ebch.1905

Frank, E., Swartz, H. A., & Boland, E. (2007). Interpersonal and social rhythm therapy: An intervention addressing rhythm dysregulation in bipolar disorder. *Dialogues in Clinical Neuroscience, 9*(3), 325–332.

Furukawa, Y., Sakata, M., Yamamoto, R., Nakajima, S., Kikuchi, S., Inoue, M., Ito, M., Noma, H., Takashina, H. N., Funada, S., Ostinelli, E. G., Furukawa, T. A., Efthimiou, O., & Perlis, M. (2024). Components and delivery formats of cognitive behavioral therapy for chronic insomnia in adults: A systematic review and component network meta-analysis. *JAMA Psychiatry, 81*(4), 357–365. https://doi.org/10.1001/jamapsychiatry.2023.5060

Galanter, M. (1988). Zealous self-help groups as adjuncts to psychiatric treatment: A study of recovery, Inc. *American Journal of Psychiatry, 145*(10), 1248–1253.

Gellatly, J., Bower, P., Hennessy, S., Richards, D., Gilbody, S., & Lovell, K. (2007). What makes self-help interventions effective in the management of depressive symptoms? Meta-analysis and meta-regression. *Psychological Medicine, 37*(9), 1217–1228. https://doi.org/10.1017/S0033291707000062

Glick, B., & Gibbs, J. C. (2011). *Aggression replacement training* (3rd ed.). Research Press.

Goldstein, A. P., Glick, B., & Gibbs, J. C. (1998). *Aggression replacement training* (Rev ed.). Research Press.

Gottman, J. M. (1994a). *Why marriages succeed or fail: And how you can make yours last*. Simon & Schuster.

Gottman, J. M. (1994b). *What predicts divorce?* Lawrence Erlbaum Associates.

Gottman, J. M., & Silver, N. (1999). *The seven principles for making marriage work*. Crown.

Greenberg, M. T. (2023). Evidence for social and emotional learning in schools. *Learning Policy Institute*. https://doi.org/10.54300/928.269

Gregory, R. J., Schwer Canning, S., Lee, T. W., & Wise, J. C. (2004). Cognitive bibliotherapy for depression: A meta-analysis. *Professional Psychology: Research and Practice, 35*(3), 275–280. https://doi.org/10.1037/0735-7028.35.3.275

Griffin, K. W., Botvin, G. J., Scheier, L. M., & Diaz, T. (2023). Long-term effects of a school-based drug abuse prevention program: Thirteen-year follow-up of participants in a randomized trial. *Addictive Behaviors, 139*, 107601.

Gualano, M. R., Bert, F., Martorana, M., Voglino, G., Andriolo, V., Thomas, R., Gramaglia, C., Zeppegno, P., & Siliquini, R. (2017). The long-term effects of bibliotherapy in depression treatment: Systematic review of randomized clinical trials. *Clinical Psychology Review, 58*, 49–58. https://doi.org/10.1016/j.cpr.2017.09.006

Guinness World Records. (2024). *Best selling first-person shooter (FPS) video game series*. https://www.guinnessworldrecords.com/world-records/87955-best-selling-first-person-shooter-fps-videogame-series

Haidt, J. (2024). *The anxious generation: How the great rewiring of childhood is causing an epidemic of mental illness*. Penguin Press.

Hansen, W. B., Dusenbury, L., Bishop, D., & Derzon, J. H. (2023). Evaluation of the D.A.R.E. Keepin' it REAL elementary curriculum: Short-term behavioral outcomes among 5th-grade students. *Journal of Primary Prevention, 44*(2), 123–145.

Hasselle, A. J., Srisarajivakul, E. N., Garza, A., et al. (2025). Effectiveness of dialectical behavior therapy skills groups as a universal school-based social emotional learning program for adolescents: A systematic review and meta-analysis. *Adolescent Research Review, 10*, 641–656. https://doi.org/10.1007/s40894-025-00259-1

Haynes, P. L., Gengler, D., & Kelly, M. (2016). Social rhythm therapies for mood disorders: An update. *Current Psychiatry Reports, 18*(8), 75. https://doi.org/10.1007/s11920-016-0712-3

Hesketh, I., Cooper, C. L., & Ivy, J. (2021). Workplace mental health interventions: A systematic review of best practices and organizational outcomes. *Occupational Medicine, 71*(5), 215–223.

Huesmann, L. R., Dubow, E. F., Boxer, P. B., Bushman, B. J., Smith, C. S., Docherty, M. A., & O'Brien, M. J. (2021). Longitudinal predictions of young adults' weapons use and criminal behavior from their childhood exposure to violence. *Aggressive Behavior, 47*(6), 621–634. https://doi.org/10.1002/ab.21984

Hornsveld, R. H., Kraaimaat, F. W., Muris, P., Zwets, A. J., & Kanters, T. (2015). Aggression replacement training for violent young men in a forensic psychiatric outpatient clinic. *Journal of Interpersonal Violence, 30*(18), 3174–3191. https://doi.org/10.1177/0886260514555007

Ijaz, S., Davies, P., Williams, C. J., Kessler, D., Lewis, G., & Wiles, N. (2020). Psychological therapies for treatment-resistant depression in adults: A Cochrane review. *BJPsych Advances, 26*(5), 254–256. https://doi.org/10.1192/bja.2020.50

Jamison, C., & Scogin, F. (1995). The outcome of cognitive bibliotherapy with depressed adults. *Journal of Consulting and Clinical Psychology, 63*(4), 644–650. https://doi.org/10.1037/0022-006X.63.4.644

Joling, K. J., van Hout, H. P., van't Veer-Tazelaar, P. J., van der Horst, H. E., Cuijpers, P., van de Ven, P. M., & van Marwijk, H. W. (2011). How effective is bibliotherapy for very old adults with subthreshold depression? A randomized controlled trial. *The American Journal of Geriatric Psychiatry, 19*(3), 256–265. https://doi.org/10.1097/JGP.0b013e3181ec8859

Jung, H., Seo, E., Han, E., Henderson, M. D., & Patall, E. A. (2020). Prosocial modeling: A meta-analytic review and synthesis. *Psychological Bulletin, 146*(8), 635–663. https://doi.org/10.1037/bul0000235

Kaur, S., & Kaur, S. (2021). Self-esteem and reactive aggression: An EMG biofeedback training approach. *American Journal of Applied Psychology, 10*(2), 49–54. https://doi.org/10.11648/j.ajap.20211002.13

Kaya, F., & Buzlu, S. (2016). Effects of aggression replacement training on problem solving, anger and aggressive behaviour among adolescents with criminal attempts in Turkey: A quasi-experimental study. *Archives of Psychiatric Nursing, 30*(6), 729–735. https://doi.org/10.1016/j.apnu.2016.07.001

Kazdin, A. E., Siegel, T. C., & Bass, D. (1992). Cognitive problem-solving skills training and parent management training in the treatment of antisocial behavior in children. *Journal of Consulting and Clinical Psychology, 60*(5), 733–747. https://doi.org/10.1037/0022-006x.60.5.733

Kazdin, A. E. (1997). Parent management training: Evidence, outcomes, and issues. *Journal of the American Academy of Child and Adolescent Psychiatry, 36*(10), 1349–1356.

Kellam, S. G., Mackenzie, A. C., Brown, C. H., Poduska, J. M., Wang, W., Petras, H., & Wilcox, H. C. (2011). The good behavior game and the future of prevention and treatment. *Addiction Science & Clinical Practice, 6*(1), 73–84.

Kellam, S. G., Wang, W., Mackenzie, A. C., Brown, C. H., Ompad, D. C., Or, F., Ialongo, N. S., Poduska, J. M., & Windham, A. (2014). The impact of the good behavior game. *Prevention Science, 15*(Suppl 1), S6–S18. https://doi.org/10.1007/s11121-012-0296-z

Kelly, J. F., Humphreys, K., Ferri, M., & Alcoholics Anonymous Work Group. (2020). Alcoholics Anonymous and other 12-step programs for alcohol use disorder. *Cochrane Database of Systematic Reviews, 3*, CD012880. https://doi.org/10.1002/14651858.CD012880

Kelly, J. F., Humphreys, K., & Bergman, B. G. (2023). Who affiliates with SMART recovery? A comparison of individuals with alcohol use disorder choosing SMART recovery, Alcoholics Anonymous, both, or neither. *Journal of Substance Abuse Treatment, 150*, 109056.

Kelly, J. F., Bergman, B. G., & Humphreys, K. (2026). Comparative recovery outcomes in a self-selected cohort attending SMART recovery, Alcoholics Anonymous, both, or neither: Six-month findings from a naturalistic longitudinal study. *Journal of Substance Abuse Treatment, 158*, 212–224.

Khanna, M. S., & Kendall, P. C. (2010). Computer-assisted cognitive behavioral therapy for child anxiety: Results of a randomized clinical trial. *Journal of Consulting and Clinical Psychology, 78*(5), 737–745. https://doi.org/10.1037/a0019739

Kindred, R., Bates, G. W., & McBride, N. L. (2022). Long-term outcomes of cognitive behavioural therapy for social anxiety disorder: A meta-analysis of randomised controlled trials. *Journal of Anxiety Disorders, 92*, 102640. https://doi.org/10.1016/j.janxdis.2022.102640

Kraft, M. A. (2019). Interpreting effect sizes of education interventions. *Educational Researcher, 49*(4), 241–253.

Kymissis, E., & Poulson, C. L. (1990). The history of imitation in learning theory: The language acquisition process. *Journal of the Experimental Analysis of Behavior, 54*, 113–127.

Lamb, H. R., & Zusman, J. (1982). The seductiveness of primary prevention. In F. Perlmutter (Ed.), *New directions for mental health services: Mental health promotion and primary prevention* (pp. 19–30). Jossey-Bass.

Laugeson, E. A., & Frankel, F. (2010). *Social skills for teenagers with developmental and autism spectrum disorders: The PEERS treatment manual*. Routledge.

Laura and John Arnold Foundation. (2017). *Social programs that work review: Evidence summary for parent management training–the oregon model*. https://evidencebasedprograms.org/document/parent-management-training-the-oregon-model-evidence-summary/

Lee, A. H., & DiGiuseppe, R. (2018). Anger and aggression treatments: A review of meta-analyses. *Current Opinion in Psychology, 19*, 65–74. https://doi.org/10.1016/j.copsyc.2017.04.004

Leurent, M., Ducasse, D., Courtet, P., et al. (2024). Efficacy of 12-step mutual-help groups other than Alcoholics Anonymous: A systematic review and meta-analysis. *European Archives of Psychiatry and Clinical Neuroscience, 274*, 375–422. https://doi.org/10.1007/s00406-023-01667-x

Lewinsohn, P. (1986). *Control your depression*. Simon & Schuster.

Lewinsohn, P. M., Antonuccio, D. O., Steinmetz, J. L., & Teri, L. (1984). *The coping with depression course: A psychoeducational intervention for unipolar depression*. Castalia Publishing Company.

Lewis, C., Pearce, J., & Bisson, J. I. (2012). Efficacy, cost-effectiveness and acceptability of self-help interventions for anxiety disorders: Systematic review. *British Journal of Psychiatry, 200*(1), 15–21. https://doi.org/10.1192/bjp.bp.110.084756

Liu, Y., Zhao, S., Zhang, X., Zhang, X., Liang, T., & Ning, Z. (2025). The effects of imagery practice on athletes' performance: A multilevel meta-analysis with systematic review. *Behavioral Sciences, 15*(5), 685.

Lopata, C. (2003). Progressive muscle relaxation and aggression among elementary students with emotional or behavioral disorders. *Behavioral Disorders, 28*(2), 162–172.

Low, A. (1950). *Mental health through will-training*. Willett Publishing Company.

Mahoney, J. L., Durlak, J. A., & Weissberg, R. P. (2018). An update on social and emotional learning outcome research. *Phi Delta Kappan, 100*(4), 18–23.

Marsiglia, F. F., Kulis, S., Ayers, S. L., Nuño-Gutiérrez, B. L., & Martínez-Rodríguez, R. (2025). Cultural adaptation and dissemination of the Spanish-language Keepin' it REAL substance-use prevention program in Latin America: Implementation and early outcomes. *Prevention Science, 26*(1), 45–60.

Mayhew, S. L., & Gilbert, P. (2008). Compassionate mind training with people who hear malevolent voices: A case series report. *Clinical Psychology & Psychotherapy, 15*(2), 113–138. https://doi.org/10.1002/cpp.566

McKendree-Smith, N. L., Floyd, M., & Scogin, F. R. (2003). Self-administered treatments for depression: A review. *Journal of Clinical Psychology, 59*(3), 275–288. https://doi.org/10.1002/jclp.10128

Mead, N., MacDonald, W., Bower, P., Lovell, K., Richards, D., Roberts, C., & Bucknall, A. (2005). The clinical effectiveness of guided self-help versus waiting-list control in the management of anxiety and depression: A randomized controlled trial. *Psychological Medicine, 35*(11), 1633–1643. https://doi.org/10.1017/S003329170500560X

Mei, Z., Cai, C., Luo, S., Zhang, Y., Lam, C., & Luo, S. (2024). The efficacy of cognitive behavioral therapy for insomnia in adolescents: A systematic review and meta-analysis of randomized controlled trials. *Frontiers in Public Health, 12*, 1413694. https://doi.org/10.3389/fpubh.2024.1413694

Meichenbaum, D. (2001). *Treatment of individuals with anger-control problems and aggressive behaviors: A clinical handbook*. Institute Press.

Melin, K., Skarphedinsson, G., Thomsen, P. H., Weidle, B., Torp, N. C., Valderhaug, R., Højgaard, D. R. M. A., Hybel, K. A., Nissen, J. B., Jensen, S., Dahl, K., Skärsäter, I., Haugland, B. S., & Ivarsson, T. (2020). Treatment gains are sustainable in pediatric obsessive-compulsive disorder: Three-year follow-up from the NordLOTS. *Journal of the American Academy of Child and Adolescent Psychiatry, 59*(2), 244–253. https://doi.org/10.1016/j.jaac.2019.01.010

Merikangas, K. R., He, J. P., Burstein, M., Swanson, S. A., Avenevoli, S., Cui, L., Benjet, C., Georgiades, K., & Swendsen, J. (2010). Lifetime prevalence of mental disorders in U.S. adolescents: Results from the National Comorbidity Survey Replication—Adolescent Supplement (NCS-A). *Journal of the American Academy of Child and Adolescent Psychiatry, 49*(10), 980–989. https://doi.org/10.1016/j.jaac.2010.05.017

Meuret, A. E., Ritz, T., Treanor, M., Dour, H. J., & Craske, M. G. (2022). *Positive affect treatment for depression and anxiety: Client workbook*. Oxford University Press.

Molteni, F., & Biolcati, F. (2023). No religion in Europe? A multilevel study of religious decline and individual disaffiliation. *Journal of Contemporary Religion, 38*(1), 1–20. https://doi.org/10.1080/13537903.2023.2165514

Naylor, E. V., Antonuccio, D. O., Litt, M., Johnson, G. E., Spogen, D. R., Williams, R., McCarthy, C., Lu, M. M., Fiore, D. C., & Higgins, D. L. (2010). Bibliotherapy as a treatment for depression in primary care. *Journal of Clinical Psychology in Medical Settings, 17*(3), 258–271. https://doi.org/10.1007/s10880-010-9207-2

Newmark, G. (1976). *This school belongs to you and me*. Hart Publishing.

Nordin, M., & Almén, D. (2017). Long-term unemployment and violent crime. *Empirical Economics, 52*, 1–29. https://doi.org/10.1007/s00181-016-1068-6

Norcross, J. C. (2006). Integrating self-help into psychotherapy: 16 practical suggestions. *Professional Psychology: Research and Practice, 37*(6), 683–693. https://doi.org/10.1037/0735-7028.37.6.683

Norris, L. A., & Kendall, P. C. (2020). A close look into *Coping cat*: Strategies within an empirically supported treatment for anxiety in youth. *Journal of Cognitive Psychotherapy, 34*(1), 4–20. https://doi.org/10.1891/0889-8391.34.1.4

O'Dean, S. M., Summerell, E., Harmon-Jones, E., Creswell, J. D., & Denson, T. F. (2025). The associations and effects of mindfulness on anger and aggression: A meta-analytic review. *Clinical Psychology Review, 118*, 102584. https://doi.org/10.1016/j.cpr.2025.102584

Palagini, L., Aquino, G., Alfi, G., Massoni, L., Gambini, M., Miniati, M., Marazziti, D., Riemann, D., Gemignani, A., & Geoffroy, P. A. (2024). CBT-I for prevention and early intervention in mental disturbances: A systematic review and meta-analysis. *Sleep Medicine, 124*, 650–658. https://doi.org/10.1016/j.sleep.2024.10.033

Patterson, G. R. (1982). *Coercive family process*. Castalia Publishing Company.

Patterson, G. R., Forgatch, M. S., & Degarmo, D. S. (2010). Cascading effects following intervention. *Development and Psychopathology, 22*(4), 949–970. https://doi.org/10.1017/S0954579410000568

Plante, T. G., Feldman, D. B., Ge, J., & Cortese, A. (2025). A randomized controlled trial assessing the psychological benefits of a daily examen-based practice. *Journal of Religion and Health, 64*(2), 1239–1256. https://doi.org/10.1007/s10943-025-02259-w

Prescott, A. T., Sargent, J. D., & Hull, J. G. (2018). Meta-analysis of the relationship between violent video game play and physical aggression over time. *Proceedings of the National Academy of Sciences of the United States of America, 115*(40), 9882–9888. https://doi.org/10.1073/pnas.1611617114

Qaseem, A., Kansagara, D., Forciea, M. A., Cooke, M., Denberg, T. D., & Clinical Guidelines Committee of the American College of Physicians. (2016). Management of chronic insomnia disorder in adults: A clinical practice guideline from the American College of Physicians. *Annals of Internal Medicine, 165*(2), 125–133. https://doi.org/10.7326/M15-2175

Rector, N. A., & Beck, A. T. (2012). Cognitive behavioral therapy for schizophrenia: An empirical review. *The Journal of Nervous and Mental Disease, 200*(10), 832–839. https://doi.org/10.1097/NMD.0b013e31826dd9af

Reid, M. J., Webster-Stratton, C., & Beauchaine, T. P. (2001). Parent training in head start: A comparison of program response among African American, Asian American, Caucasian, and Hispanic mothers. *Prevention Science, 2*(4), 209–227. https://doi.org/10.1023/a:1013618309070

Ritterband, L. M., Thorndike, F. P., Ingersoll, K. S., Lord, H. R., Gonder-Frederick, L., Frederick, C., Quigg, M. S., Cohn, W. F., & Morin, C. M. (2016). Effect of a web-based cognitive behavior therapy for insomnia intervention with 1-year follow-up: A randomized clinical trial. *JAMA Psychiatry, 74*(1), 68–75. https://doi.org/10.1001/jamapsychiatry.2016.3249

Rohde, P., Clarke, G. N., Mace, D. E., Jorgensen, J. S., & Seeley, J. R. (2004). An efficacy/effectiveness study of cognitive-behavioral treatment for adolescents with comorbid major depression and conduct disorder. *Journal of the American Academy of Child and Adolescent Psychiatry, 43*(6), 660–668. https://doi.org/10.1097/01.chi.0000121067.29744.41

Sanders, M. R., Baker, S., & Turner, K. M. (2012). A randomized controlled trial evaluating the efficacy of triple P online with parents of children with early-onset conduct problems. *Behaviour Research and Therapy, 50*(11), 675–684. https://doi.org/10.1016/j.brat.2012.07.004

Santos, R. M. S., Mendes, C. G., Sen Bressani, G. Y., de Alcantara Ventura, S., de Almeida Nogueira, Y. J., de Miranda, D. M., & Romano-Silva, M. A. (2023). The associations between screen time and mental health in adolescents: A systematic review. *BMC Psychology, 11*(1), 127. https://doi.org/10.1186/s40359-023-01166-7

Schonert-Reichl, K. A., Oberle, E., Lawlor, M. S., Abbott, D., Thomson, K., Oberlander, T. F., & Diamond, A. (2015). Enhancing cognitive and social–emotional development through a simple-to-administer mindfulness-based school program for elementary school children: A randomized controlled trial. *Developmental Psychology, 51*(1), 52–66.

Scogin, F., Hamblin, D., & Beutler, L. (1987). Bibliotherapy for depressed older adults: A self-help alternative. *The Gerontologist, 27*(3), 383–387. https://doi.org/10.1093/geront/27.3.383

Scogin, F., Jamison, C., & Davis, N. (1990). Two-year follow-up of bibliotherapy for depression in older adults. *Journal of Consulting and Clinical Psychology, 58*(5), 665–667. https://doi.org/10.1037/0022-006X.58.5.665

Scogin, F., Jamison, C., & Gochneaur, K. (1989). Comparative efficacy of cognitive and behavioral bibliotherapy for mildly and moderately depressed older adults. *Journal of Consulting and Clinical Psychology, 57*(3), 403–407. https://doi.org/10.1037/0022-006X.57.3.403

Seligman, M. E. P. (1998). *Learned optimism: How to change your mind and your life*. Vintage Books.

Shi, B., & Cheung, A. C. K. (2024). Cross-age tutoring and its effects on academic achievement and social development: A systematic review and meta-analysis, Educational Research Review, *41*, 100559.

Shure, M. B., & Spivack, G. (1979). Interpersonal cognitive problem solving and primary prevention: Programming for preschool and kindergarten children. *Journal of Clinical Child Psychology, 8*(2), 89–94. https://doi.org/10.1080/15374417909532894

Shure, M. B., & Spivack, G. (1980). Interpersonal problem solving as a mediator of behavioral adjustment in preschool and kindergarten children. *Journal of Applied Developmental Psychology, 1*(1), 29–44. https://doi.org/10.1016/0193-3973(80)90060-X

Shure, M. B., & Spivack, G. (1982). Interpersonal problem-solving in young children: A cognitive approach to prevention. *American Journal of Community Psychology, 10*(3), 341–356. https://doi.org/10.1007/BF00896500

Smeijers, D., Bulten, E., Buitelaar, J., & Verkes, R. J. (2018). Treatment responsivity of aggressive forensic psychiatric outpatients. *International Journal of Offender Therapy and Comparative Criminology, 62*(12), 3834–3852. https://doi.org/10.1177/0306624X17747052

Smith, G. Pew Research Center. (2025). *Religious landscape study: Religion holds steady in America*. https://www.pewresearch.org/religion/2025/12/08/religion-holds-steady-in-america/. https://doi.org/10.58094/dkgp-6k90

Smith, N. M., Floyd, M. R., Scogin, F., & Jamison, C. S. (1997). Three-year follow-up of bibliotherapy for depression. *Journal of Consulting and Clinical Psychology, 65*(2), 324–327. https://doi.org/10.1037/0022-006X.65.2.324

Stallard, P., Simpson, N., Anderson, S., Carter, T., Osborn, C., & Bush, S. (2005). An evaluation of the FRIENDS programme: A cognitive behaviour therapy intervention to promote emotional resilience. *Archives of Disease in Childhood, 90*, 1016.

Stallard, P., Simpson, N., Anderson, S., & Goddard, M. (2008). The FRIENDS emotional health prevention programme: 12 month follow-up of a universal UK school based trial. *European Child & Adolescent Psychiatry, 17*, 283–289.

Stallard, P., Skryabina, E., Taylor, G., Phillips, R., Daniels, H., Anderson, R., & Simpson, N. (2014). Classroom-based cognitive behaviour therapy (FRIENDS): A cluster randomised controlled trial to prevent anxiety in children through education in schools (PACES). *The Lancet. Psychiatry, 1*(3), 185–192. https://doi.org/10.1016/S2215-0366(14)70244-5

Strayhorn, J. M. (2005). Pilot study of telephone tutoring in reading skills. *Perceptual and Motor Skills, 101*, 505–509.

Suinn, R. M. (1972). Behavior rehearsal training for ski racers. *Behavior Therapy, 3*(3), 519–520.

Taylor, J. L., & Novaco, R. W. (2022). Treatment for anger, aggression, and violence. In W. R. Lindsay & J. L. Taylor (Eds.), *The Wiley handbook on offenders with intellectual and developmental disabilities: Research, training, and practice* (pp. 248–271). John Wiley & Sons.

Tinson, A. (2020). What the quality of work means for our health. *The Health Foundation*. https://www.health.org.uk/reports-and-analysis/briefings/what-the-quality-of-work-means-for-our-health

Ungerleider, S., & Golding, J. M. (1991). Mental practice among Olympic athletes. *Perceptual and Motor Skills, 72*, 1007–1017.

Valente, T. W., Okamoto, J., Alexander, J., & Dyal, S. R. (2022). A randomized controlled trial of the D.A.R.E. Keepin' it REAL curriculum in elementary and middle schools. *Prevention Science, 23*(4), 623–637.

Van Ryzin, M. J. (2016). A systematic review of family-based interventions for preventing adolescent substance use. *Journal of Child and Family Studies, 25*(5), 1430–1444.

Vigna-Taglianti, F. D., Galanti, M. R., Burkhart, G., Caria, M. P., Vadrucci, S., Faggiano, F., & EU-Dap Study Group. (2014). "Unplugged," a European school-based program for substance use prevention among adolescents: Overview of results from the EU-Dap trial. *New Directions for Youth Development, 2014*(141), 67–112. https://doi.org/10.1002/yd.20087

von Brachel, R., Hirschfeld, G., Berner, A., Willutzki, U., Teismann, T., Cwik, J. C., Velten, J., Schulte, D., & Margraf, J. (2019). Long-term effectiveness of cognitive behavioral therapy in routine outpatient care: A 5- to 20-year follow-up study. *Psychotherapy and Psychosomatics, 88*(4), 225–235. https://doi.org/10.1159/000500188

Webster-Stratton, C. (1998). Preventing conduct problems in head start children: Strengthening parenting competencies. *Journal of Consulting and Clinical Psychology, 66*(5), 715–730. https://doi.org/10.1037/0022-006x.66.5.715

West, S. L., & O'Neal, K. K. (2004). Project D.A.R.E. Outcome effectiveness revisited. *American Journal of Public Health, 94*(6), 1027–1029.

Wilcox, H. C., Petras, H., Brown, H. C., & Kellam, S. G. (2022). Testing the impact of the whole-Day good behavior game on aggressive behavior: Results of a classroom-based randomized effectiveness trial. *Prevention Science, 23*(6), 907–921. https://doi.org/10.1007/s11121-022-01334-y

Wolpe, J. (1969). *The practice of behaviour therapy*. Penguin Books.

Wu, T., Gao, X., & Chen, M. (2021). Workplace interventions to promote employee mental health: A systematic review of best practices. *Occupational Health Science, 5*(3), 345–372.

Xia, J., Merinder, L. B., & Belgamwar, M. R. (2011). Psychoeducation for schizophrenia. *Cochrane Database of Systematic Reviews, 2011*(6), CD002831. https://doi.org/10.1002/14651858.CD002831.pub2

Yuan, S., Zhou, X., Zhang, Y., Zhang, H., Pu, J., Yang, L., Liu, L., Jiang, X., & Xie, P. (2018). Comparative efficacy and acceptability of bibliotherapy for depression and anxiety disorders in children and adolescents: A meta-analysis of randomized clinical trials. *Neuropsychiatric Disease and Treatment, 14*, 353–365. https://doi.org/10.2147/NDT.S152747

Zion Market Research. (2026). *FPS game market size, share, industry analysis, trends, growth, 2032*. https://www.zionmarketresearch.com/report/fps-game-market.

Chapter 9
The Obstacles and the Promise

Abstract We are enthusiastic about what thorough, widespread psychoeducation *could* do for society. The skills that are required for psychological health are known, and the sorts of influences that make these skills better or worse are also known. We can, and we should, envision ways of teaching all people these skills, starting from a very early age, and continuing such teaching for many years, or for a lifetime. With not only competence learning, but also much greater attention to creation and cultivation of mental-health-friendly environments, the biological vulnerabilities to psychopathology, which are also quite important, would almost certainly do significantly less damage. However, optimism about what psychoeducation *could* do does not translate into a prediction of what it *will* do. A problem is that although our technology for broadcasting stories that could be models of psychological health is unparalleled, human beings tend to focus on stories of violence and psychopathology. Another problem is that when many people get involved in the psychoeducational effort, as they must, a certain fraction will be abusive or just incompetent. Still, the job is too large to relegate only to licensed health care professionals. Psychoeducation can become a mission shared by schools, workplaces, families, religious institutions, community organizations, governments, communications media, authors, and individuals. If this mission is pursued with maximum quantity and quality of effort, the results could go beyond reduced prevalences of disorders; there could be a society where happiness and peace prevail.

Keywords Promise of psychoeducation · Scalability · Obstacles · Exploitation of children · Mass media · Motivation for mental health

The question we have taken on in this book goes far beyond what is usually thought of as the bailiwick of the health care system. We are not just dealing with trying to reduce the number of cases of certain types of disorders. With mental health defined in terms of the skills necessary to produce happiness in oneself and others, the collective "mental health" of a society is tantamount to how desirable that society is to

J. M. Strayhorn, Jr. et al., *The Promise of Psychoeducation in Relieving the Societal Burden of Psychopathology*, SpringerBriefs in Modern Perspectives on Disability Research, https://doi.org/10.1007/978-981-92-0922-4_1

live in. The issue is improving the human condition, making life better for all of those who live it.

We've made the case that the skills people need to get, in order to achieve those goals, are teachable and learnable. As we've enumerated in great detail earlier, they include favorable habits of self-talk, of decision-making, of emotional responses, of relationship development, and particularly of being kind to one's fellow human beings. They include those of creating positive environments in which people can flourish. And they are teachable, not primarily by didactic lecturing, but by at least ten methods of influence that are constantly operative among humans, for better or for worse.

While acknowledging the benefits of psychotropic medication, we've raised doubt that much improvement of the collective well-being of society is likely to result from psychopharmacology. Part of the problem is the bluntness and lack of focus with which drugs work: for example, there will likely never be a drug that specifically alters the brain to make it possible to play the piano, nor a drug that specifically injects some particular assertive but non-defensive responses to criticism into the behavioral repertoire. But we already have the nonpharmacological means to produce just those brain alterations, called learning.

We've been very favorable toward psychotherapy as a cooperative venture aimed at goals of mental health. But we've despaired of the possibility that the collective mental health of society will be much affected if the burden of improving psychological skills is turned over to licensed professionals who must document every session, and who are incentivized to see one "identified patient" at a time—the numbers just don't work out. There are too many of us who need improvement in psychological skills (approximately all of us), too few psychotherapists, not enough money allocatable to the psychotherapy enterprise, and not enough people who are able to and want to spend their time in this way. But psychotherapy, and the psychoeducational offshoots of it, have demonstrated over and over the crucial and wonderful fact that mental health skills can be learned.

Let's indulge in a whimsical fantasy. Suppose it became certain that unless the average level of human proficiency in a certain set of skills reached a certain level by a certain time, the world would explode and most life would be wiped out. Conversely, if the specified level of proficiency were attained, the world would be a very happy place for almost all people to dwell in. What would be the best course of action? Surely it would be to use widely what we already know about imparting those skills, to study continually how to impart the skills more effectively, to start teaching those skills early in life, to make it as pleasant as possible for people to learn them, to monitor effectiveness regularly, and to celebrate greatly the improvements along the way toward the magic threshold. We would use the mass media to present positive models of the skills and the steps to attain them. We would enlist as enormous a teaching force as possible, and encourage people to teach each other.

If one considers that conflict resolution, nonviolence, kindness, and development of positive relations are mental health skills, and that human civilization now possesses enough weapons to destroy itself, the whimsical fantasy may not be far from the truth. The Bulletin of the Atomic Scientists (2026) at the time of this writing has set the clock closer to the "midnight" of doom than it has ever been since this metric was started in 1947. Of course, universal teaching of psychological skills is neither the only way nor the most quick-acting way of preventing the destruction of society; and there are compelling reasons to teach psychological skills in addition to prevention of doomsday. Still, the whimsical fantasy reminds us that society is not presently collaborating on something like a "moon shot" or "Manhattan Project" to improve its own psychological skills, despite all the work we have cited. In the words of Albert Einstein (1946), "The unleashed power of the atom has changed everything save our modes of thinking and we thus drift toward unparalleled catastrophe."

To produce the most optimistic scenario, we would extrapolate from the psychoeducational efforts we have discussed, many of which managed to bring forth statistically significant results from only a few hours invested. If such results could be obtained by a one-time intervention of a few hours, what results could be obtained by ongoing intervention, over years, as is the case with reading, writing, or mathematics work? (An estimate of one hour of work, for each of 180 school days, in kindergarten through 12th grade, yields a total of 2340 hours of "time on task.")

But difficulties in achieving, in real life, anywhere close to such amounts of time on task is a major obstacle to the promise of psychoeducation. Current educational systems, in the USA at least, often seem driven by an inertia of rules constraining the time available for psychoeducation, despite the fact that psychological skills work can be carried out simultaneously with work on reading and writing skills.

Another major obstacle to the attainment of the psychologically skilled society is the competition posed by mass media, many of which (most obviously shooter games, but extending much more generally) seem constructed so as to provide maximum practice in violence, anger, lack of empathy, and the quest for dominance. The hours of participation in these dwarf those of most psychoeducational interventions. A major challenge to humanity is to make fantasy rehearsal of prosocial actions as appealing as fantasy rehearsal of anger and killing now is.

Another major obstacle is that the task of protecting against abuse and exploitation of learners by teachers can be formidable. The Boy Scouts of America was bankrupted by sex abuse lawsuits (Prince, 2022); Scouting organizations in other countries also took major hits. The Catholic Church in the USA has paid out over 5 billion dollars in settlements for sex abuse lawsuits, and the problem is not limited to the USA (Schlumpf, 2025). Denominations other than Catholicism have been affected (Public Broadcasting System, 2019). For all these organizations, the financial damage is minor in comparison to the loss of trust, and the loss of membership. The vision of people making a massive cooperative effort to teach psychological skills must unfortunately be tempered by massive efforts at monitoring the personnel so as to preclude predatory exploitation.

So, a caveat is that quality control is crucial and in itself laborious. Nonetheless, the mission is clearly too large to be relegated to licensed health care professionals. The mission of psychoeducation must be shouldered by schools, workplaces, families, religious institutions, community organizations, governments, communications media, authors, and individuals.

Motivation for increasing psychological skills in children appears to be very high. The Pew Research Center (Minkin & Horowitz, 2023) found that mental health worries topped the list of parents' concerns for their children: 36% were somewhat worried about anxiety or depression, and 40% were extremely or very worried. Another Pew Research Center survey of teachers (Lin et al. 2024) reported that 48% of teachers listed anxiety and depression as a major problem for their students; 49% reported the behavior of students at their school as fair or poor (not good or excellent); 68% have experienced verbal abuse; 40% have experienced violence from a student; and 52% would not advise a young person to become a teacher. Thus, at least with respect to the mental health of children and adolescents, the two groups that are around them the most, i.e., parents and teachers, seem to have the will to bring about improvements. Is it true that "Where there's a will, there's a way"?

A major purpose of this book has been to argue that there is already a way, and it is high-quality psychoeducation, delivered in large doses over many years. Larson (1984) has called this a "new paradigm": "When psychological skills and knowledge are in the hands of the public, our collective psychological IQs will be raised to the point that individuals need not struggle in isolation to solve problems that are universally experienced. No longer will they need to 'reinvent the wheel' each time they face life crises: they will be able to draw on the collective problem-solving wisdom of an entire culture." The obstacles to implementing this option are very formidable. We are not able to predict whether human society will ever be able to implement such a program. But we do feel able to predict that if such a program were thoroughly implemented, the result would be a major improvement, not only in mental health, but in the human condition. And we are tremendously gratified to have been able to document many concrete and significant steps in the right direction.

References

Bulletin of the Atomic Scientists. (2026). *It is now 85 seconds to midnight*. https://thebulletin.org/doomsday-clock/

Einstein, A. (1946, May 25). Atomic education urged by Einstein. *The New York Times*, p. 13.

Larson, D. (1984). *Teaching psychological skills: Models for giving psychology away*. Brooks/Cole. Available at https://www.scribd.com/doc/73492620/Dale-Larson-Teaching-Psychological-Skills-Models-for-Giving-Psychology-Away

Lin L., Parker K., & Horowitz J., Pew Research Center. (2024). *What's it like to be a teacher in America today?* https://www.pewresearch.org/social-trends/wp-content/uploads/sites/3/2024/04/ST_24.04.04_teacher-survey_report.pdf

Minkin, R., & Horowitz, J. M., Pew Research Center. (2023). *Parenting in America today*. https://www.pewresearch.org/social-trends/2023/01/24/parenting-in-america-today

Prince, M. (2022). The battle of bankruptcy: A look at the Boy Scouts sex abuse case. *University of Illinois Chicago Law Review.*. https://lawreview.law.uic.edu/news-stories/the-battle-of-bankruptcy-a-look-at-the-boy-scouts-sex-abuse-case

Public Broadcasting System. (2019). 3 of U.S.'s biggest religious denominations in turmoil over sex abuse, LGBT policy. https://www.pbs.org/newshour/nation/3-big-us-churches-in-turmoil-over-sex-abuse-lgbt-policy
Schlumpf, H. (2025). Catholic Church sex abuse crisis. *Encyclopaedia Brittannica.*. https://www.britannica.com/topic/Catholic-Church-Sexual-Abuse-Crisis

MIX
Papier aus verantwortungsvollen Quellen
Paper from responsible sources
FSC® C105338

If you have any concerns about our products,
you can contact us on
ProductSafety@springernature.com

In case Publisher is established outside the EU,
the EU authorized representative is:
Springer Nature Customer Service Center GmbH
Europaplatz 3, 69115 Heidelberg, Germany

Printed by Libri Plureos GmbH
in Hamburg, Germany